P9-DBL-258

MASTER YOUR
METABOLISM

THE 3 DIET SECRETS TO NATURALLY BALANCING
YOUR HORMONES FOR A HOT AND HEALTHY BODY!

JILLIAN MICHAELS

WITH MARISKA VAN AALST

FOREWORD BY CHRISTINE DARWIN, M.D.

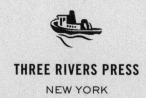

THREE RIVERS PRESS

NEW YORK

The information in this work is in no way intended as medical advice or as a substitute for medical counseling. The information should be used in conjunction with the guidance and care of your physician. Consult your physician before beginning this program as you would any weight-loss or weight-maintenance program. Your physician should be aware of all medical conditions that you may have, as well as the medications and supplements you are taking. As with any weight-loss plan, the information here should not be used by patients on dialysis or by pregnant or nursing mothers.

Published in the United States by Three Rivers Press, an imprint of the Crown Publishing Group, a division of Random House, Inc., New York.
www.crownpublishing.com

THREE RIVERS PRESS and the Tugboat design are registered trademarks of Random House, Inc.

Originally published in hardcover in the United States by Crown Publishers, an imprint of the Crown Publishing Group, a division of Random House, Inc., New York, in 2009.

Library of Congress Cataloging-in-Publication Data

Michaels, Jillian.
Master your metabolism / Jillian Michaels.
p. cm.
Includes bibliographical references.
1. Weight loss—Endocrine aspects. 2. Metabolism—Regulation. I. Title.

RM222.2.M483 2009
613.2'5—dc22   2008050510

ISBN 978-0-307-45074-6
eISBN 978-0-307-45097-5

Printed in the United States of America

Book design by Ruth Lee-Mui
Cover photograph © by Joseph Puhy

10 9 8 7 6 5 4 3 2 1

First Paperback Edition

To my baby sister, Lauren, for being the hope in my heart.
I'm so filled with pride. Watching you grow, blossom, and flourish
has inspired me to be a better woman.
This book, in title, is about mastering your body and your health,
but ultimately it's about mastering your life.
You are the master of your destiny. Shoot for the stars. Stop at nothing.
Don't forget the power you hold within you.
Thrive.

ACKNOWLEDGMENTS

I want to give special thanks to my editor and friend, Heather Jackson, for her vision and unwavering support. Mariska van Aalst, my brilliant partner in crime, thank you for your patience, blood, sweat, and tears. Andy Barzvi, thanks for helping me make this book happen. Thanks to Dr. Christine Darwin, who provided the foreword as well as consulted on the condition-specific plans offered later in the book. To my team of Giancarlo Chersich, Steve Blatt, Tammy Munroe, David Markman, Kevin Huvane, Jonathan Swaden, and Lisa Shotland, without you I am nothing. My assistant, Janet Graham, for putting up with me and indulging my neurosis. My mother, for her unconditional love.

Everyone at Crown, NBC, Waterfront Media, Icon, Lionsgate, Majesco, Nintendo, and KFI, for helping me build a brand with integrity and purpose. *Thank you, all . . . for everything!*

CONTENTS

PART THREE: THE MASTER TOOLS

FOREWORD

BY CHRISTINE DARWIN, M.D.

As an endocrinologist, I often meet people who are looking for an explanation for their fatigue or weight gain that is associated with their hormones and metabolism.

This unique book addresses hormones in an easy-to-read format, and Jillian Michaels explains, in a superb way, her own personal life experiences about how she turned her mistakes into learning opportunities for others. The book reflects not only Jillian's passion for advocating a healthy lifestyle that includes physical fitness, but also her commitment to helping readers learn essential information about hormones, diet, and health.

This simple guide answers many of the most frequently asked questions, especially in the areas of hormones and weight issues. It's a book for everyone, because it addresses people of all ages who want to incorporate healthy eating with a balanced lifestyle. *Master Your Metabolism* even serves as a helpful guide to parents who are concerned about their children being at hormonal risk, especially in today's world, where childhood obesity is skyrocketing into an epidemic.

In addition to those patients with legitimate hormonal concerns, I also meet otherwise healthy people who insist on taking some sort of hormones on a regular basis because they erroneously believe they will achieve some favorable effects in overcoming a weight or metabolic problem. As a doctor treating many patients with similar conditions, I advise against putting more hormones into your body to deal with such issues. In fact, hormones will not help. Instead, they pose a danger of altering your natural hormone production. Additional hormones can cause long-term negative effects on your body that can lead to dependence for the rest of your life.

Your body needs regular medical checkups. You have to pay close attention to what is going on inside, just like you sort the mail everyday or "declutter" your room and living spaces. We don't accept spam or junk mail on our computers because it is of no good use to us. The same is true when it comes to harmful and toxic products that make their way into our bodies. We have to throw them away. They are no good to us. They need to be removed regularly, otherwise they will cost us space, time, and eventually will dominate the healthy aspects of our lives.

Some products are healthy just like those documents we hold on to and file away. Healthy nutrients and good habits such as exercising at least thirty minutes three to four times a week are the kind of things we want to keep. Exercise gives us a sense of reward and helps us to reap enormous benefits even with minimal amount of weight loss. Exercise harmonizes with your hormones to optimize your internal biochemistry and helps you to reclaim your body once again.

Jillian's book illustrates the environmental challenges we face daily and how stress influences our bodies emotionally and physically. It shows us how to avoid those challenges and get ahead of the stress so we can restore and reclaim a healthy body. The important work within these pages also emphasizes how vital it is to balance our psychological, hormonal, nutritional, and physical exercise to achieve a long, healthy, and rewarding life.

As you read this book, you will receive the necessary tools to understand how hormones work so you can begin to recognize and remove all toxic influences that can creep into your life. Also, as you read and learn, you will want to consult your physician to correct any hormone issues so you can reclaim your body.

Congratulations! You are about to embark on an amazing journey that will inspire you to eliminate toxins and rebalance your life with healthy habits as you take charge of your body.

—Christine Darwin, M.D., F.A.C.P., F.A.C.E.
  Associate Professor of Medicine
  David Geffen School of Medicine at University of California,
  Los Angeles (UCLA)

INTRODUCTION:
TAKE BACK YOUR METABOLISM

WHY HORMONES MATTER—TO ALL OF US

I could have called this book *The Evolution of a Health and Fitness Guru*. Why? Because after seventeen years of work in the fitness field—seventeen years of studying with the world's top doctors in sports medicine, nutrition, endocrinology, and antiaging—this is everything I've learned. Yes, this is what it has all been leading up to: *Master Your Metabolism*, my total approach to optimal weight and optimal health.

This book is the distillation of my entire journey in health, from childhood binge eater to weight-loss guru. I've been at this for almost two decades, but what I've learned in the past few years completely changed my body and my life.

My first book, *Winning by Losing*, centered on the psychological and behavioral aspects of losing weight. In that book, I focused on how to get yourself into a frame of mind so you'd be ready to lose weight. (If you're just getting started with an exercise program, and want an approachable plan, you might want to check it out, too.)

My second book, *Making the Cut*, was my ode to fitness. It is a physical fitness regimen designed to get rid of those last ten pounds—the hard way! It is ruthless, but very effective (insert evil laugh here). It gets you shredded, blasts the problem areas, like muffin tops and saddlebags, and helps you prep for that big event or party where you want to look your best. (If you have only a few pounds to lose and want to get fit fast, its thirty-day plan will work for you.)

This book, however, has nothing to do with exercise.

Surprised?

I know, that's not what you expect to hear from me. I've gone on and on in the past about the benefits of exercise. And you and everyone else know it's good for you. So that's not the purpose of this book.

And it's not a calorie-counting book either.

I know what you're thinking: that after being such a tyrant about exercise and watching calories, I've finally gone soft, right? Wrong!

Master Your Metabolism is, first and foremost, a diet book. My very first diet book. And let me tell you—if you practice what I'm preaching here, it will change your life, in more ways than just being skinny. I'm talking about adding years of quality to your life.

We all know that fad diets are a thing of the past, and that the no-carb, no-fat crazes of the eighties and nineties are scientific laughingstocks and pop-culture dinosaurs. Welcome to the future—this is the era of genome mapping, stem-cell research, and nutrigenomics (the study of how food communicates with our genes). Yes, calorie counting and exercise are very important, but they are not the whole story. Underneath the dieting and workout programs are the little messengers that carry information from your body to your brain and vice versa. These "little messengers" are your hormones.

What do hormones have to do with anything? Let me explain. If I were to ask you what your metabolism is, what would you say? I bet you would answer, "The way my body burns calories."

If so, you would be wrong. That's one of the key things your metabolism *does*. But do you know what it *is*?

The answer is *hormones*! Your metabolism *is* your biochemistry.

Some hormones tell you you're hungry, some tell you you're full. When you eat, hormones tell your body what to do with that food, whether to store it or burn it as fuel. And when you exercise, hormones tell the body how to move and consume energy stores, and how to boost or shut down different parts of the body. Hormones control almost every aspect of how we gain weight—and how we can lose it.

Maybe right now you're thinking, "I'm a guy—I don't have to worry about hormones." Or, "If this book is about hormones, it's not for me—I'm twenty years away from menopause."

That's what I thought, too! I'm only thirty-four—what could my weight possibly have to do with my hormones? But guess what: Whether you're a girl or a guy, whether you're young or old, your weight has *everything* to do with your hormones. Whether you want to lose the freshman fifteen, the postbaby belly, or the beer gut, your hormones determine whether you'll succeed or fail. And right this minute, your hormones—and by definition your metabolism—are being set up to fail. Without you even knowing it, your hormones have been hijacked by toxin-filled, nutritionally deficient, stress-dominated systems—endocrine disruptors—that cause obesity and disease. These systems lurk in surprising places, but they ultimately disrupt our hormone function and cause hormone imbalances—in *all* of us.

That's why I designed *Master Your Metabolism*: to identify these catalysts of obesity and disease, cut them out at the roots, and create a state of optimal health where the body and mind function at maximal efficiency. Together, we'll target and eliminate these endocrine disruptors and replace them with the hormone-positive systems that make you healthy, happy, and skinny, no matter how old you are.

Synthesizing what the science of endocrinology can teach you about your metabolism, your eating habits, and your weight, *Master Your Metabolism* gives you a clear-cut plan that makes the latest research work for you and your individual biochemistry. And this complete lifestyle plan will help you not only lose that weight but keep it off once and for all.

THE SECRET TO PERMANENT WEIGHT LOSS: HORMONAL HARMONY

The endocrine system is sometimes compared to an orchestra. Each hormone is like an instrument. Playing together, in tune, they sound amazing. But what happens if, right in the middle of a concert, the violin suddenly goes wildly astray, twanging away? And then the clarinet starts shrieking? And then the pianist can't keep a steady pace?

They would sound like crap, right?

It's exactly the same with your metabolism. Your body can't work the way it's supposed to if any of your hormones is out of tune. Once one loses the beat, they all follow. That's why, when your hormones are off note, you can't just focus on one hormone at a time—you have to work to get them all in tune and playing in the right key again.

You've probably heard the words *cortisol, growth hormone* (or *HGH*), *insulin,* and *leptin*—especially being thrown around on weight-loss infomercials at one A.M. Am I right? Well, those words are the names of hormones, and those hormones dramatically affect your weight and your health.

So the weight-loss products that target them must work, right? Hardly. Thing is, those bunk "treatments" focus on only one hormone at a time (if they even work at all), which is a very incomplete and misleading picture.

Unlike those infomercials, instead of trying to isolate one hormone at a time—which is totally impossible—this book is about how you can naturally optimize *all* of your hormones. And how you can do it without taking dangerous or expensive drugs.

Our hormones—all of them—are influenced by millions of things in our diet and environment, from processed foods to pesticides to lack of sleep to excess stress. Any disruption will kick one hormone into overdrive and another into hibernation mode. When the normal function of one hormone gets thrown off, that imbalance creates another, and another, and another. Way too often, these chronic imbalances make you fat—even when you are ruthless and meticulous about calorie counting and burning.

I want to teach you that you can get your hormones in check simply by changing your habits in the grocery store and at the kitchen table. We're going to dig deep here and **remove** all the toxic crap that damages your endocrine system, turns on your fat-storing hormones, and causes you to gain weight. Then we'll **restore** the nutrients that speak directly with your fat-burning hormones to nudge them back to most favorable levels. Finally, we'll **rebalance** the energy going into and out of your body, so that your metabolism works for you as a fat-burning machine, instead of against you, storing fat and stealing energy.

When your hormones are at their optimal levels, your body functions at peak efficiency:

Your metabolism starts jammin'.
You look a lot better.
Your body maintains a healthy weight without much conscious effort.
Your belly flattens.
Your skin is clear and radiant; your hair and nails are strong and shiny.
Your eyes are bright.
Your senses are keen, not dulled.
You don't suffer from excessive hunger or crazy cravings.
You get cut and lean.

You have energy to burn.

You live a longer, healthier life.

If you've seen me on television or heard me on the radio, you know that I am like a dog with a bone—I do not give up. I have perfected this plan to work for everyone. And I've done it the way I've worked to help every one of my clients and *Biggest Loser* contestants—through careful attention to detail and relentless persistence. I've taken all the latest cutting-edge research and personally tested it to make sure I could offer the healthiest, most effective eating and lifestyle program possible.

Believe it or not, I've fine-tuned this plan to the point where I can eat two thousand calories a day, and hit the gym for 2 to 3 hours a week (gotta love those grueling work schedules!), and still manage to maintain my physique.

Sounds crazy? It's possible for you, too.

The best part is, I've done all this work so now you don't have to!

I know you have a hectic and full life. I know you hate plans that make you count and chart and obsess about minute details. Forget all that. I may be tough in the gym, but I'm going to make it easy on you on this diet. Just pull up a seat at the table and enjoy.

In this book, you'll learn how to

- Optimize *all* the hormones that are necessary to lose weight
- Fix your metabolism so it works for you, not against you
- Choose foods and habits that trigger weight-loss hormones
- Avoid foods and habits that trigger weight-gain hormones
- Learn which foods work together and how to cook them for maximum endocrine benefit
- Prepare fast, hormone-balancing meals with items already in your kitchen
- Eat incredibly well on a few bucks a day
- Correct biochemical dysfunction with relaxation techniques
- Detoxify your environment so that hormones readjust and weight drops off
- Enjoy fresh foods that can prevent cancer, heart disease, depression, diabetes, and other diet and lifestyle-related diseases
- Dramatically increase energy levels and potentially lengthen your life by many years

As you work your way through the book, you can follow this program either as general guiding principles or as a specific, prescribed weight-loss plan. I'll break it down in as much detail as you need—do it all or just take the major lessons and go on your way. It's your call.

I want you to begin to see everything that we're up against, and start making choices that follow the major tenets of this plan. Do that, and you'll take back control of your hormones, restart your metabolism, and get it revving faster than it ever has. *Because, bottom line, this is not a book about being thin to be healthy. It's about being healthy to be thin.*

Ready? Let's go.

PART 1

THIS IS YOUR METABOLISM ON HORMONES

CHAPTER 1

LET ME GUESS— IS THIS WHAT'S HAPPENING TO YOU?

How I Came to Realize My Hormones Were Totally Screwed Up

I tried putting the pieces together every which way, but the story was always the same.

Doctor after doctor, study after study, test after test, told me this very scary fact: In my quest to be "skinny," I had abused my body for years and years. Rather than getting thinner, I'd succeeded only in aging myself, screwing up my hormone levels, and teaching my body to be *fatter*.

Now, before you say, "Jillian, give me a break—look at your body," hang on a sec. If you've seen me on TV, you know I'm not a slacker. (I guess you don't get called "TV's toughest trainer" for being a softy.) True, I have logged many hours in the gym. I have literally worked my butt off for the body that I have.

But that's my point: Despite all of that work, my body still wasn't responding the way it should have, which is when I realized I was missing a piece of the puzzle. Today, it kills me to realize that I could've done half the work to get the body I have, had I just known then what I know now.

Now I know that the solution to living happily and healthily is hormone balance—not an impossible regimen that sucks the joy out of life. When I learned how to eat and live in a way that balanced and optimized levels of key hormones, most of my weight-loss battle was won before I even set foot in the gym.

Let me guess. Do you have

- a scale that's stuck, no matter how little you eat or how much exercise you do?
- a sagging energy level that seems only to be getting worse?
- skin that's starting to turn sallow or wrinkle excessively—and you're not even past forty?
- skin that's constantly breaking out—and you're decades past adolescence?
- moods that peak and trough unpredictably?
- a monthly cycle that drives you (and everyone around you) absolutely nuts?
- crushing fatigue that doesn't improve, no matter how much sleep you get?
- a burned-out, slightly "crispy" feeling that you can't shake?
- Have you lost and gained the same five, ten, twenty pounds, over and over?
- Or, more likely, have you lost and gained steadily more each time, losing ground, getting more and more hopeless?

I did, too. All that and more. I knew something was wrong, but I couldn't figure it out—I thought I was going insane. That's when I started digging into the field of endocrinology—the branch of medicine that deals with hormones—and slowly but surely realized (with no small amount of horror) that I was bringing a lot of this on myself.

But it took me a really, *really* long time to figure that out—and I don't want that to happen to you.

A NATION OF HORMONE IMBALANCE

When I look around, I know I'm not alone. There are a *lot* of screwed-up endocrine systems out there. The statistics tell the story:

- 24 million Americans have diabetes (1 in 4 don't even know it yet).
- 57 million Americans have prediabetes.
- 1 in 4 people have metabolic syndrome.
- 1 in 10 people have an underactive thyroid gland.
- 1 in 10 women have polycystic ovarian syndrome (PCOS).
- 1 in 13 women have severe PMS.

That's before we even start talking about the 33 million women barreling straight toward menopause. Boomers, sure, but I'm talking about the first Gen Xers, too. Then add on another 33 million men headed for andropause, aka "male menopause," which, yes, really does exist.

All of these conditions are caused by hormonal imbalance. Some are the predictable result of aging; some are brought on by genetic predisposition. But what's the most common symptom of an out-of-whack endocrine system?

Excess body fat, plain and simple.

Obesity—not to mention premature aging and disease—is caused by hormonal imbalances that gradually wear down the endocrine system until it is tricked into packing on pounds. And once your metabolism thinks you want to put on weight, it does all it can to accommodate you.

That's why two out of three of us are overweight, and one in three of us have become obese.

And that's why I wrote this book.

Together, we're going to reeducate you and your metabolism so that your body becomes a naturally vibrant, invigorated fat-burning machine.

▶ THE GREAT HORMONAL FAKE-OUT

Any and every body function you can imagine is controlled by your hormones. From minute to minute, your biochemistry tries to maintain homeostasis—a sense of balance—in your body. In addition to helping all the systems of your body—your kidneys, gut, liver, fat, nervous system, reproductive organs—communicate with one another, your hormones have another enormous job. Whenever your body interacts with millions of external variables—the contents of your meal, the time of day, the intensity of your workout—your endocrine system responds, releasing hormones to help you balance your blood sugar, go to sleep, burn fat, or build muscle.

The only problem is that sometimes those external variables shoot way off the charts, and your hormones don't know which way is up. They try to help your body regain balance, but in the face of unhealthy foods, environmental toxins, or too much stress, they begin to overreact and overcompensate. And that's when the problems start.

Too many stressful deadlines spike belly-fat-creating cortisol. Synthetic estrogens in the environment assault the body from every corner, and fake out your testosterone. Too many missed nights of sleep make fat-burning growth hormones dip low. Skipped lunches make the hunger hormone ghrelin jump. Addictions to sugared sodas stop satiety (fullness) hormones like leptin from working.

These dramatic hormonal shifts weren't part of your body's original plan. So the unpredictable fluctuations start to wear down your body's natural regulatory processes. Your endocrine system no longer understands what balance looks like. It stops responding the way it should. Your organs take a beating; your glands burn out. You get hypothyroid, leptin-resistant, and insulin-resistant.

And then you gain weight.

That's why we need to get your body back in balance. And that's what this book will do. I'm going to give you all the tools you need to regain control of your body's biochemistry. Together, we're going to press the reset button on your metabolism and retrain your hormones, so that instead of gaining, you can start losing weight—a lot of it.

▶ WHAT'S AT STAKE

There's evidence of a national endocrine meltdown everywhere. More Americans are overweight than ever before—72 million of us. Obesity is the second leading cause of preventable death. Only the act of lighting known carcinogens on fire and repeatedly inhaling them into your lungs— aka smoking—beats it out for the deadliest spot.

People who are obese are 50 to 100 percent more likely to die earlier than people of normal weight. They also have a higher rate of many debilitating and/or deadly conditions:

- Arthritis
- Atherosclerosis (hardening of the arteries)
- Cancer (especially cancer of the pancreas, liver, kidney, endometrium, breast, uterus, and colon, and possibly leukemia and lymphoma)
- Congestive heart failure
- Coronary heart disease
- Crushing depression
- Devastating social stigma
- Gallbladder disease
- Gout
- Heart attacks
- High blood pressure
- High cholesterol
- High triglycerides
- Respiratory problems
- Sleep apnea
- Stroke
- Thicker heart walls
- Type 2 diabetes

I wish I were making this stuff up to scare you, but I'm not. We've all read the headlines. We know there are supposedly many reasons why this is happening: twenty thousand cable TV channels, super mega cheeseburgers, processed foods, fifty-mile commutes to work, seventy-hour workweeks.

But there are other reasons that no one seems to be talking about. What about the chemicals in our air, water, cosmetics, clothes? How about the weed killer on our neighbors' lawns? How about the plastic that's invaded every corner of our world?

We've demonized our "supersize me" habits for a long time. But there are many other environmental, dietary, and societal factors that have come into play only in the past thirty years, and a vast number of them disrupt our hormones and switch off our metabolisms.

I have watched so many people I love go down the path of hormone-induced early death. You know that guy—maybe you *are* that guy—with a barrel of heart-attack fat strapped onto his waist. Or that woman who finds a lump in her breast at twenty-eight. Or the kid who gets diagnosed with "adult onset" type 2 diabetes before he's allowed to see a PG-13 movie.

This last one is such a heartbreaker for me. The diagnosis rate for diabetes has shot up 40 percent in the past decade. What the heck is going on here? Why are our hormones spinning so out of control, and how are we ever going to stop them?

Clearly, there is only one way. We have to wake up and realize that every bite we take and every lifestyle choice we make matters. Not just for calories or fat or carbs, but because those bites or choices tell our bodies how to react. With bite after bite, sip after sip, breath after breath—when we pick the wrong foods or surround ourselves with toxic chemicals, each moment of consumption tells our hormones to do things that, consciously, we would never want them to do.

We have to learn how our modern food supply and toxic world interact with our hormones. We have to understand exactly *how* they make us overweight and sick. That's the only way we can set it right again. And that is what *Master Your Metabolism* is all about.

CONFESSIONS OF A FORMER FAT KID

Just how far have we strayed from the path of natural hormone balance?

Pretty damn far, actually. And I know, because for many years of my life, I was way, way off it myself.

I'm going to tell you what happened to me, how my hormone levels got entirely messed up, not because it's so unusual, but because many of the same things have probably happened to you and everyone you know. Without realizing it, even a fitness guru can have all her hard work undermined by out-of-whack hormones—so how does a teacher or a salesman or a stay-at-home mom stand a chance?

It all began when I was a total chubster.

I may look ripped now, but I spent my early years constantly struggling with excess weight.

Part of what started it all was living with my dad. My dad was an addict. And food was just one of his addictions. He was also very likely hypothyroid, although none of us knew that at the time. But his addiction to food and his genetic predisposition for being overweight definitely was transferred to me.

> French fries are one of the three most common vegetables consumed by infants 9 to 11 months of age.

I'd hang out with my dad at home when my mom was going to night school studying to be a psychologist. Food was the only way that he knew how to show affection or relate to me. He would make huge buckets of popcorn and we would watch *Buck Rogers* together. Or we would make pizzas together. He even got into making us homemade ice cream.

If we left the house, we'd go out to our special chicken schwarma place, or the burrito place we liked. Food became one of the only connections I had with my dad.

But my issues with food didn't all come from Dad. My mom, who was always skinny, would sometimes use food as a reward. I was an only child, and if my parents were both out, they would leave me with a sitter. I *hated* being with a sitter. So before the sitter got there, they'd take me to the bakery and say, "Pick whatever you want." Or my dad would just order me a napoleon because that was his favorite. And on the way out of the bakery, I could have a rum ball, an extra little baked confection. Those things still have such a bizarre emotional connection for me, it's scary.

My mom knew I missed her when she went to work, so before she left for the day, she'd say, "What would you like from the vending machine?" As soon as she got home, she'd bring me my Twix bar. I had an elaborate Twix-eating ritual: First, I'd carefully eat the entire caramel layer off the top of the cracker. Then I'd dunk the cracker in a glass of milk. These food rituals were a comfort to me. They were steady, consistent, reliable—and eventually very destructive.

That's how it always was in my family, as far back as I can remember. Once when I was three years old, my parents were having a conversation about separating. They gave me a bag of Cheetos and put me in the kitchen while they argued in the next room. I remember sitting at the kitchen table alone in front of a huge bag of Cheetos, wondering, "What does this mean for me?" No brothers or sisters at the time. No real support, but the Cheetos were there for me. The food kept me company. It gave me something to look forward to that I knew was consistent and wouldn't let me down.

Sad, huh?

My parents ultimately got divorced when I was twelve. Not coincidentally, that was really the pinnacle of my weight gain. Everything was falling apart for me. I was skipping school, failing in my classes, experimenting with the contents of my parents' liquor cabinet—doing all kinds of bad things, dangerous things.

I started stealing my mom's car after school—now, bear in mind, I was *twelve*. I'd get home in the afternoon while she was still at work, and grab her spare keys. I would take out the Jeep

THE ROOTS OF FAT, PART 1: IT'S (PARTIALLY) IN THE FAMILY

Consider these elements of the family environment that are associated with an increased risk of developing obesity:

- Mother's weight: By the age of 6, kids born to overweight mothers are 15 times more likely to be obese than kids born to normal-weight mothers.
- Breast-feeding: Numerous studies link breast-feeding to lowered chance of childhood obesity. Some experts estimate that bottle-fed babies have a 15 to 20 percent greater chance of being obese than breast-fed babies.
- Television: Every hour of television teens watch increases their risk of developing obesity by 2 percent. Reducing television viewing to 1 hour a week could cut the number of obese teens by almost one-third.
- Family meals: A survey of 8,000 kids found that those who didn't eat many meals with their family but watched a lot of TV were more likely to become overweight by the third grade.
- No outdoor play: If those kids also lived in unsafe neighborhoods that didn't allow for outdoor play, they'd be fat by kindergarten.
- Parental control: If parents are very controlling about what kids eat, their kids never develop the ability to self-regulate their intake and will likely become overweight.
- Dieting too early: Boys and girls who are encouraged to diet are three times more likely to be overweight five years later, due to increased binge eating, skipped breakfasts, or other unhealthy attempts to lose weight.
- Poverty: Lower income combined with any of these factors increases the risk of obesity dramatically. I believe that toxins in our environment target the most vulnerable people: poor children whose parents can afford only the most widely available, genetically modified, pesticide-laced, corn- and soy-based processed food.

Cherokee and race around the neighborhood like a crazy person. I was very lucky that I didn't kill someone, including myself.

While I was out in the car, I'd hit my fast-food regulars. It started with a Taco Bell run: two bean and cheese burritos with no onions and extra cheese. Then it was two bean and cheese burritos with no onions and extra cheese and a taco. Then, three bean and cheese burritos with no onions and extra cheese and a taco supreme—and, come to think of it, sure, throw in the cinnamon sticks and a Coke.

Or, after school, I would order a Domino's pizza, go sit on the roof of my house, eat the whole thing. Or I would get a bag of Cheetos and eat the entire bag while I watched *Punky Brewster* or *The Facts of Life*—I would just sit on the couch and gain weight and be miserable.

Around this time, I started having dreams that I was a POW in a war zone. I became obsessed with movies about the Vietnam War, and I literally started to believe I was a reincarnated POW. The day my parents' divorce was finalized, I kicked a hole in the wall.

I was twelve years old, five feet tall, and weighed about 175 pounds. (In other words, I was two inches shorter and 55 pounds heavier than I am now.)

My mom took a good look at me and realized she had to act—and fast. She took me to a therapist, but thankfully she also recognized that I needed a physical outlet to release my anger and frustration.

And that's when martial arts saved my life.

ENTER EXERCISE—AND POWER

At the time, my mom was dating this guy whose nephews were taking martial arts from a teacher who was a bit unconventional, to say the least. I was intrigued. At some level, my mom sensed it would be the right thing for me, but sending your kid to this instructor was kind of like sending her off to military school. He did not mess around.

His name was Robert David Margolin and he taught out of a dojo in his garage in the Calabasas Hills. Robert created a hybrid style, a mix of aikido and Muay Thai called Akarui-Do. In essence, he was one of the first mixed martial arts pioneers. He became a sort of father figure to me—but he was definitely a renegade.

He was very extreme, and I loved it. It felt more real to me than a tamer, more conventional approach would have. I guess I'm just drawn to extremes. (You might have guessed this about me already.)

The men at that small dojo became like brothers to me. They were all dedicated to their health and were driven, spiritual, and focused. Because I looked up to them so much, I began to realize that all the other stuff I was doing—the drinking, the ditching school, and basically making a mess of my life—was not cool. *This* was cool to me. I wanted to be just like these people. I wanted to impress them.

So, what was it Rob said to me that finally got my ass in gear? Here is the story. I believe everyone who is serious about changing their lives has one of these—I call it "the rock-bottom moment." It's the epiphany that ultimately drives you toward change—no matter what.

One day while I was waiting for my lesson, I was standing there, scarfing down my bag of Cheetos. Robert came out to get me, took one look at the bag, and threw me out of the studio. "You're wasting my time," he said to me. "And until you're ready to pick up what I'm laying down, you're wasting your own time, but I actually *value* my time. So get out." I felt the blood drain out of my body. He saw how stunned I was. "If you want to take this seriously, and take yourself seriously, then come back and I can help you out." And he shut the door in my face.

Robert's message to me, which became my guiding philosophy since that moment, was: The entire journey to health is about power. The definition of power, in my opinion, is learning how to make your dream a reality.

Let me tell you a little secret: I don't love working out. Sometimes I do, but it's rare. I couldn't care less if somebody has six-pack abs or buns of steel. Don't get me wrong, if you have that, good for you. But fitness is about so much more for me.

I use fitness to empower people. It makes people feel strong and confident and potent, and that strength transcends into other parts of life.

And now I understand that it's the same with your diet and other aspects of your lifestyle. Once you make the decision to take control of what goes into your body, you're able to harness that power. By recognizing that forces outside of your body have been disrupting your internal biochemistry, and taking steps to optimize your hormones, you're tapping in to that same power, reclaiming it for yourself.

The day Robert kicked me out of his studio, I was fourteen. I'd been there just over a year. I suddenly realized how far I'd come. I'd gone from

being the fat kid in school who couldn't take her eyes off the ground—
the one who ate lunch in Mrs. Cronstad's office every single day because
I was so afraid to show my face in the school yard—to being the kid who
would walk down the hall and look people in the eye and think, "You can't
talk to me like that—I just broke two boards with my right foot. Bring it."

I couldn't risk losing that power again.

Working with Robert turned me around psychologically, gave me con-
fidence, and showed me a way of life that I valued and that would help
me achieve my dreams. He helped me realize that the stronger I was
physically, the more potent I was as a human being.

But I still didn't understand one key thing. Robert didn't care whether
I was skinny. I did. But he couldn't have cared less. He wanted me to eat
a healthy diet to take care of my body, but I didn't really get *that* part of
his message until many years later.

▶ HOT YOUNG THING

By seventeen, I was a certified fitness trainer. And I was vain.

I was a young woman living in Los Angeles. Naturally, I wanted to look
good. I was voracious about it. There was nothing that I didn't read or
know about. I had every trade magazine, from *Muscle & Fitness* to *Shape*.
I read every diet book, tried every fitness craze. I saw what worked and
what didn't.

I was studying Navy SEAL training, poring over books about Bruce Lee
and Israeli SWAT team methods. I spent hours and hours in the gym,
doing the craziest stuff—I was doing plyometrics and high-intensity workouts a decade before they hit the mainstream. I would go to the gym and
hang upside down by one gravity boot or do one-arm pull-ups like it was
nothing.

People at the gym would see me and think, "What the heck is this girl
doing?" Then a couple of them started coming up to me and asking me to
train them. That's how my career as a trainer began—people wanted me
to teach them all the crazy stuff I was doing to myself.

I wasn't even thinking of making a career out of it. I was already bartending at night. (With a fake ID, I might add—still a bit of a rebel. Some
things never change.) I was making really good money for a teenager. I
didn't need the extra money. I never looked for clients. I just thought,

"Well, I'm doing this for me, but if you want me to, sure, I'll train you. What the heck? Could be fun."

Of course at that point I had no idea this would be my destiny, helping people change their bodies and their lives through fitness and health. I was still going through my own saga, my own continuing struggle with my weight.

The average American woman has tried to lose weight at least 10 times.

I was obsessed with finding the right ways to burn fat, not just for my clients but for me. For example, for a while, I followed the prevailing belief that the most effective way to burn fat was to work out on an empty stomach. Then I had the chance to talk to a biochemist about it and came to find out that it was exactly the wrong thing to do because your body will metabolize its own muscle tissue! Scratch that, move on to the next thing.

I did the same thing with my diet. I experimented with Pritikin, Atkins, Blood Type, pH, Paleolithic, vegetarianism, food combining—even the dreaded Master Cleanse—you name the diet, I went on it. Why? Because I wanted to be skinny!

For a full decade, I treated my body like I was a lab rat. How could I have dreamed that all these extreme experiments were messing with my hormones? All I cared about was never going back to being the fat kid, and frankly, I didn't care how I got the results I was looking for.

Working in the gym, reading up on all the latest diet research, I was totally in my element, loving life. But then, somehow, I got lost in cubicle land for a few years.

▶ THE RAT RACE CLAIMS ANOTHER RAT

Have you ever made a choice in your life that seemed like a mild course correction but turned into a major detour? That's what happened to me, and it took me *years* to get back on track.

I was happily training people during the day and bartending at night, not thinking so much about the future, just having fun. But then I started taking flak from a guy I was dating. "Jillian, you're twenty-three," he said. "You live in Los Angeles. You can't be a *trainer* [as if he were saying *drug dealer*] for the rest of your life. You need to get serious. You need to get a career."

From that point on, I thought, "Oh, I guess being a trainer isn't a real career." Probably the saddest part was that I didn't think of training people as a career precisely *because* I liked it so much. Something so fun couldn't be work, right? Tragic.

I told myself I needed to get serious and find an "adult job." So I went to work at a major talent agency in Los Angeles.

For the next four excruciating, soul-crushing years, I burned the candle at both ends, holding down a sixty-hour-a-week desk job with sky-high stress and 100 percent butt-in-chair time. Yet even if I had to do my work-out at midnight, I was still working myself into the ground at the gym, still obsessed with health, still training—I just wasn't training anybody else. During my few off hours, I was still voraciously devouring every diet out there: Oh, are we on the Zone now? Hold on, now we're doing metabolic typing, is that it? What's this South Beach thing—is this the way? Because it was always a constant battle with my weight, my body, my health. Day in and day out, I was slavishly counting every last calorie.

About this time, I noticed that I had a kind of blotchy brown spot on my face that wouldn't go away. I went to the dermatologist. Turned out I had melasma, also known as "the mask of pregnancy," extreme hyper-pigmentation on the face that's often caused by high levels of estrogen and progesterone. My dermatologist looked at it and said, "We could do a peel to lighten it."

I thought, "Peel it? Hang on—why am I getting it in the first place?" I'd never been pregnant and I wasn't on birth control pills. What was going on?

I didn't have time to think about it. Stressed to the gills, living on processed (i.e., *fake*) diet foods, artificial sweeteners, sugar alcohols, and caffeine, I was forcing myself through my days, gutting it out through a sheer naked addiction to Diet Coke—I'd have a six-pack, or *more*, every day.

From the outside, my job was really glamorous. I didn't wait in line at restaurants. People "knew" me. I worked in Hollywood, for goodness' sake. I thought I was a big shot.

> People who report job stress have a 73 percent higher chance of developing obesity and a 61 percent higher chance of developing abdominal fat than people who report none.

But in reality, I hated my job, hated what I was doing. Every morning I would wake up and basically want to scream. I felt like my life had no meaning.

You know that saying, "Things

are always darkest before the dawn"? My darkest point was getting caught in a power struggle between two agents. I knew something terrible about one of them, something he'd been doing that would definitely get him fired, if not sued. The stress of knowing this information was too much for me. (Plus, to be honest, I really couldn't stand him.) So when the upper management pulled me in to question me about what he'd done, I spilled it. The whole story. I told them what he'd done and how he'd done it.

You see where this story is going, don't you?

The agent renegotiated his contract. They fired me. And now I had a mortal enemy for life.

What happened next was straight out of *You'll Never Eat Lunch in This Town Again*. He blackballed me all over town. I couldn't get a job. I couldn't even get off the couch. I just sat there thinking, "I wasted four years of my life killing myself for no reason, being miserable. And for what?"

At a certain point, I had no choice—I had to make money. A friend hired me at a sports fitness place to be a physical therapy assistant. I had to suck it up and work for about a tenth of my former salary, putting towels on kids who were assistants at the company that had just fired me—kids I'd sent to that gym when I was their superior at work! The whole experience was just mortifying.

And just about the best thing that ever happened to me.

A bad day for your ego is a great day for your soul.

HOME AGAIN—AND VERY CLOSE TO ANSWERS

As it turned out, that gigantic ego check was exactly what I needed. The move put me back in my element and made me humble and hungry enough to work hard again. After a long time of trying to live up to someone else's definition of success, I was back where I belonged. And happy, for the first time in years.

Within just a few months, I'd helped the center extend its offerings and open a full gym. My client list started to fill up—I was working with celebrities like Vanessa Marcil and Amanda Peet, Hollywood agents and producers, all new clients who had come to me because of my time in the entertainment industry. As I became more established, I would get to speak with these celebrities' nutritionists, dietitians, and sports medicine doctors, all the best in the business. Believe me, I never wasted a chance to pick their brains. I'd take these theories that I learned and say, "Explain Atkins to me. Where's the science behind this diet? What is it really doing?" The picture was gradually becoming clearer, but I still wasn't putting all the pieces together—especially not about what was happening in my own body.

By the following year, I had opened my own sports medicine facility in Beverly Hills, complete with three physical therapists, a physiatrist, and a chiropractor. Soon after that, I started getting calls from *Shape, Self, Redbook,* and *Marie Claire* whenever they needed an interview on a new fitness, diet, or weight-loss phenomenon.

Professionally I was rockin', and my future looked bright. But through it all, I was *still* constantly struggling to keep my weight down. The only reason I was staying in shape was because I was meticulous, and I mean *me-ti-cu-lous,* about counting calories. I was training my body rigorously for seven to eight hours a week. Even as I told my clients to drink tons of water, I was *heavily* addicted to caffeine, pounding diet sodas hourly.

> For each can of diet soft drink consumed each day, a person's risk of obesity goes up 41 percent.

God forbid I should fall off the wagon for a few days. I'd instantly gain five pounds, which would then drive me back to the grueling routine. After all the effort I'd put into learning about diet and nutrition, I just couldn't figure out why all my working out and freaky eating habits weren't doing the trick. I really thought I'd been royally screwed in the genetics department—that my metabolism just sucked, and I would never be able to have it as easy as some of my friends.

But as it turned out, the reality was that a body can handle that kind of strain for only so long before it gives out completely. Which is what happened when I joined the cast of *The Biggest Loser.*

Now, if a girl's gonna go on TV and inspire people to lose hundreds of pounds, she's gotta look good, right? That was my guiding thought as I prepared to be on camera. "I have to be ripped. Gotta make an impression," I'd tell myself, so I would severely restrict my calories to twelve hundred a day while killing myself in the gym. This was the only way to get my body in amazing shape. I had one chance to get people's attention and make an impression. I had to be in the best shape of my life—to walk the walk, you might say.

Well, I walked the walk, all right—the walk of the living dead. I was exhausted. Worked to the bone and stressed to the max.

As soon as the season ended, I went from twelve hundred calories a day to a healthy eighteen hundred, a perfectly reasonable shift for someone who worked out as hard as I did.

And I put on fifteen pounds practically overnight.

But it wasn't like I just went home and stuffed myself with pizza. I was still working out five hours a week! If I had a single glass of wine, I gained weight. Again, I had to kill myself to get it back off.

Something else was going on. This is ridiculous, I thought. Something was definitely wrong with my metabolism. It just shouldn't be this bloody hard.

FINDING THE KEYS TO THE KINGDOM

Then, right about this time, I hit the big 3-0. Funny thing about turning thirty, it really makes a person think—about the possibility of having kids, about the desire to live longer and healthier. Up until that point—and this might seem a little bit funny—I had always assumed I was going to die young.

> After age 20, basal metabolic rate drops about 2 percent per decade; after 40, it slows down 5 percent per decade.

When I got there, I realized I wasn't James Dean—I wasn't going to get the easy way out. And I didn't want it! I wanted to have a long life, to grow up and age gracefully.

The journey wasn't just about being thin anymore; it was about health and longevity, too. I wanted not just a skinny body but a healthy, happy, and long life as well.

At this point, a good friend and client of mine had been seeing an endocrinologist. I got on the phone with this doctor to discuss the health and wellness of my client, which was totally routine for me. I'd pretty much worked with the entire medical community of Los Angeles, seen or talked to every dietitian, sports medicine doctor, biochemist, chiropractor, podiatrist . . . you name it. But this was my first endocrinologist.

While talking to this doctor, I finally understood why my client wasn't seeing results. All the missing pieces of the puzzle were right in front of me. My client had hypothyroidism, which is why we couldn't get off her last fifteen pounds. She was also suffering from PCOS, which is linked to type 2 diabetes, which was also making her metabolism function at a snail's pace. *Whoa.*

I knew she had a slow metabolism, but now I knew why. And with his help, we created a diet plan to change it for her.

Incredible, I thought. I *have* to get this done to myself. "How soon can I get in there?" I asked. "Can I drive over right now?"

Eventually I did put myself at the endocrinologist's mercy. I got tested for everything from cholesterol to heavy-metal poisoning. I still remember the day I was sitting in his office when he strolled in with my results. He smiled, handed me a piece of paper, and, before I had a chance to read it, said, "How long have you been hypothyroid?"

I blinked. The paper was full of numbers in the "abnormal range" column.

"And your testosterone is really low. Have you ever been on Accutane?"

I couldn't catch my breath.

"Do you know what 'estrogen-dominant' means?"

At that point, I almost felt dizzy. All of a sudden, I had a completely plausible explanation for all the symptoms I'd ignored or denied for so many years: my facial pigmentation, my peaks and troughs of energy, and, yes, those fifteen instant pounds. The uniting factor was my *hormones*.

My fat-storing stress hormones, like cortisol, were through the roof. My fat-burning youth hormones, like growth hormone and DHEA, were plunging. I had more estrogen floating around than my body knew what to do with. My entire endocrine system was entirely whacked-out—and with it, my metabolism.

This realization was one of the greatest awakenings of my career. And from that moment on, I was unstoppable. I was totally new to this world, but I saw an avenue to fix things and make them right.

I channeled all the energy I'd previously put into slashing and burning calories into this new obsession. I began studying the science of antiaging, meeting with the best toxicology experts and endocrinologists around the country.

I started to learn about environmental toxins and their effects on the body. I got into organics. Just as I had in the gym as a teen, I dug up the most obscure research, tried it out, and saw what didn't work—and what did. I began to truly understand why I'd always struggled with my weight, and that I had made it so much harder than it should have been.

I learned that burning the candle at both ends and my unhealthy obsession with dieting and food restrictions had really done a number on my hormones and, consequently, my metabolism.

Realization #1: Since I was fourteen, my entire diet had consisted of foods with the word *free* in them: fat-free lunch meat, carb-free bread, sugar-free yogurt. In other words, nonfoods, Frankenfoods, creepy-scary processed foods. To my horror, I learned that synthetic chemicals in these "foods" talked to my cells on a DNA level. They could even switch on fat-storage genes that might have lain dormant had I just eaten an apple instead of the Apple-icious Sugar-Free Chemi-Cookies. And, naturally, all of these foods were packaged in plastics that sent out even more endocrine-disrupting messages to my body!

Realization #2: The extreme version of the "calories in, calories out" equation I'd lived and dieted by had come back to slap fat on my butt. The equation remained the same; the numbers had just gotten smaller. I suddenly saw that my years of calorie restriction had trashed my resting metabolic rate by helping deplete my already weak thyroid.

Realization #3: The Accutane I'd taken for six months in my early twenties—*six or seven years before I saw symptoms*—had possibly suppressed my testosterone levels and helped me become estrogen-dominant, which gave me those hideous splotches on my face that I'd been peeling ever since. Not to mention all the lost calorie burning from a testosterone shortage! (Now, that one really made me want to cry.)

Realization #4: I had been sleeping five hours a night while preaching to my clients to get to bed earlier. "Good sleep has been linked to weight loss," I'd tell them, as I totally ignored my own advice. Now I realized that I'd been cheating myself out of the fat-burning, muscle-building hormones that my body would've released had I actually been home in bed instead of out on the town, pounding sugar-free Red Bulls.

On and on it went—every discovery about hormone balance pointed to something that I'd gotten wrong in my diet, my supplements, my lifestyle. Finally, it all made sense. It wasn't my genetics that had screwed me; I had screwed myself by burning the candle at both ends, working myself into the ground at the gym, and living on processed diet foods, artificial sweeteners, sugar alcohols, and caffeine. What a train wreck I was.

To say that I was crushed was an understatement. How many years, how many thousands of extra hours in the gym, had I logged because I

THE ROOTS OF FAT, PART 2: IT'S (PARTIALLY) IN THE GENES

You've probably heard of a theory about the so-called thrifty gene, which researchers believe evolved to help our ancestors store fat more efficiently during lean times. People with this gene developed a type of seasonal insulin resistance that allowed more of their calories to be stored as fat during times of scarcity (such as during the winter). These fat stores could later be tapped for survival, but doing so would trigger even more fat-hoarding. (So much for thrifty—sounds downright greedy to me.)

All this fat storage was very handy in feast-or-famine times. But in America today, where we produce 25 percent more calories per person since 1970, we live in feast-feast-feast times, with nary a scarcity in sight.

So having this greedy gene would really suck, right? Well, how about having *thousands* of greedy genes? A recent report in the *British Medical Journal* suggests that more than 6,000 genes—about 25 percent of the human genome—help determine our body weight. Researchers estimate that there may be up to 10 times as many genes that *increase* body weight than decrease it.

These genes—and how they are expressed in each individual—all have different actions. Some tell us to eat more or less sugar. Some spur people to fidget in their seats, burning hundreds of excess calories a day. Some genes might predispose us to metabolism-regulating thyroid disorders. Some might cause a deficiency of the satiety hormone leptin, causing us to either underproduce it or block it.

But just because your whole family is overweight doesn't mean that is your destiny. We all can change the expression of our genes by improving our physical environment as well as our cellular environment via diet and lifestyle choices.

didn't know how to protect my hormones? How much incredibly disgusting diet food had I eaten, believing it was helping me to stay skinny—when it was really making me *fatter*?

I knew that I needed to stop seeing food as an enemy, and instead start learning about it as fuel for a long and healthy life. It was this realization that turned the light on for me. For my own sanity, I had to find a way to turn my mistakes into a learning opportunity for others. That's how I created *Master Your Metabolism*.

Once I hit upon just the right combination of elements, I started to see results very quickly. Pounds started to fall off without having to spend hours in the gym. Whereas before I would have to be meticulous and watch every single calorie that passed between my lips, now I could eat normally, not be hungry, and stop obsessing about food. I had the body I always wanted—and I felt healthier and more energetic than I had my entire life.

How did I do it? I started to recognize and appreciate how *hormones affect every single bodily process,* 24-7. Of course the food I was eating, the schedule I was keeping, and the stress I was enduring were all affecting my hormones. Through trial and error, lots of consultations with doctors and experts, and tons of reading and research, I gently nudged and massaged and tweaked my entire life to help reset those hormones and optimize their levels, so that they could function the way nature had always intended them to.

And now it's your turn to do the same.

HOW THE PLAN WORKS

I'm thirty-four, and I feel healthier than I ever have before. I don't overeat, but I live on eighteen hundred to two thousand calories a day instead of twelve hundred. I spend about five hours a week in the gym at most. I don't have to do more because my body takes care of that balance naturally. For someone who practically used calculus to track her food and exercise for years, you can't imagine how freeing that is.

I don't eat synthetic crap anymore, because it tastes like poison to me now—which it is! I don't spend hours in the gym, but when I go, I go big. I have the energy to do way more than I used to, and I feel like I've turned back the clock on my age by at least a decade.

And you can, too.

No matter how you've abused your body up until now—and I'm willing to bet you have, even if you didn't mean to—you *can* make it better. You can reboot your metabolism and optimize your hormones so your body can relearn how to incinerate fat. You can learn what foods and lifestyle habits trigger weight-loss hormones and which ones dampen weight-gain hormones. You can make changes that will turn back the clock for your body and add those extra years to the back end. And you'll do it in three simple steps.

REMOVE, RESTORE, AND REBALANCE

Most likely you've been trying to do your part to help heal the earth with the three Rs: Reduce, Reuse, Recycle? Well, we're going to heal your body's metabolism with the three Rs of hormone power: Remove, Restore, Rebalance. We're going to:

REMOVE THE ANTINUTRIENTS

We're going to get that Frankenfood out of your kitchen once and for all. We'll go through your pantry and toss all the antinutrients, the toxic processed foods and synthetic chemicals that have been screwing up your metabolism—including the ones that you thought were helping you. We'll even clean up a few of the natural foods that have a surprisingly negative impact on your hormones.

RESTORE THE HORMONE POWER FOODS

We'll add back the foods that your body needs, whole, fresh foods that naturally, instinctively optimize your hormones. We'll focus on Restoring the food groups that trigger your fat-burning hormones and blunt your fat-storing hormones. Each of these hormone power foods also builds muscle, smooths skin, increases energy, and helps prevent dangerous conditions and diseases like cancer, heart disease, high blood pressure, diabetes, metabolic syndrome, and much more.

REBALANCE YOUR TIMING AND PORTIONS

No calorie counting here. We'll create an easy-to-follow, personalized plan to help you Rebalance your food intake to maintain your blood sugar balance and energy throughout the day without hunger or cravings. You'll learn how to combine foods in ways that trigger the optimal release of hormones, making sure you get all the proper nutrients in the right ratios to support your metabolism. And to keep your body burning calories throughout the day, you'll eat almost constantly—one of my favorite aspects of the plan.

Repairing your metabolism doesn't end with your diet. One of the most surprising things about my hormonal revelation was learning the impact of the environment and lifestyle on our hormones. The newspapers have been full of stories lately about the dangers of plastics leaching estrogens into our food supply. As I talked to scientists around the world, I was shocked to learn how much broader the issue of endocrine disruption goes, both in the global environment and in our own homes. But as widespread as the problem is, I was gratified to learn that there are many, many ways to reduce our risks. That's why *Master Your Metabolism* also has a lifestyle program to help you root out and minimize as many risk factors as possible in your own life. You'll learn to:

REMOVE THE TOXINS

You won't believe how many chemicals in your water supply, house, car, office—you name it—are making you fat right now. We'll continue to detoxify our bodies by removing known endocrine disruptors from our environment wherever possible. And we'll automatically help heal the earth, one house at a time.

RESTORE THE NUTRIENTS

Everything about the modern American food supply—from industrial farming to pesticide use to overprocessing—drains our food of its natural nutrients. Once you begin to restore the hormone-optimizing nutrients, you will certainly be on the right path. But sometimes your body needs more of certain vitamins and minerals to get your metabolism to full power. In those cases, I'll address any lingering deficiencies with a few supplements to Restore critical missing nutrients to your diet.

REBALANCE YOUR STRESS LEVELS

Rebalance is the final piece of this program, but in many ways this is the most important aspect. Rest and relaxation have a greater impact on hormone balance than just about anything you can do. You may have a pristine diet, but if you're stressed-out or sleep-deprived, it's not going to make that much difference. We'll Rebalance and learn how to manage the inevitable stress in our lives (as well as reset the wake/sleep balance) to keep our stress hormones in check.

> ### MY PROMISE TO YOU—AND A REQUEST

Your body has been tricked, swindled out of health. Now we're going to make it right. But I need to ask something of you, too.

You need to be an active participant here. You need to take responsibility and understand that Uncle Sam is not looking out for you. Big food companies are not on your side. Just because pesticides are legal, just because the USDA says hormones in beef are totally safe, just because your boss says you need to be married to your job 24-7—that doesn't make it so. You cannot bury your head in the sand anymore. The faux foods and chemicals and stress are messing with you on a genetic level, altering your hormones to an unrecognizable degree, poisoning your body and killing our planet one evil dollar at a time. This is not just about your waistline—this is about saving ourselves.

To be honest, it doesn't matter if you're on board with the "save the world" portion of our program. As long as you follow the diet, whether you do it for your waistline or for the planet, I don't care. The net effect is the same—your hormones will be balanced, your waistline will be smaller, and you'll be around a lot longer to enjoy the world you helped to save. Fine with me!

Before we get to the plan, let's take a quick sec just to define our terms. We could talk all day about your metabolism, but do you really know what your metabolism is made of? We'll hit the highlights of some of the key hormones that help dictate your weight. You'll get a feel for how out of whack your hormones really are—and even *if* they are. Some people are lucky, like my friend Vanessa. (You'll hear about her in a minute.) But many, many of us have at least one hormonal imbalance that has either slowed or completely halted our ability to lose weight. In the next two chapters, we'll learn about what each hormone does, the key symptoms of imbalance in the body, and how exactly we all got stuck in this hormonal meltdown to begin with.

If you're eager to get started, go ahead and jump to chapter 4 and read about the plan first. You can even dig right in with chapter 5, "Step 1— Remove," and start cleaning out your kitchen today. A lot of people like to get started with the program while they learn about the underlying issues. That's not a bad idea—*everyone* benefits from this plan, so you might as well jump right in. We don't have a second to waste here.

But when you're done there, come on back. Because as scary as some of this information is—and it *is*—knowledge is power. Now, let's talk hormones—which ones impact our weight and how we can start pushing their levels in the right direction, today.

CHAPTER 2

MEET THE KEY PLAYERS

How Your Hormones Determine Your Metabolism

Remember how I told you my life changed the day I went to the endocrinologist?

My true "Aha!" moment actually came about two weeks later.

At first when my doctor told me my endocrine system was fried, I was stunned speechless. My brain was just spinning. But then a little part of me said, "I don't know about this. Maybe he's just trying to sell me on this whole supplementation business thing he's got going."

I enlisted the help of my best friend, Vanessa, to catch him out.

Vanessa is one of those annoyingly, effortlessly thin women. And did I mention she's drop-dead gorgeous? She is five years older than me, but I've seen her wolf down more food than her lithe little frame could possibly burn off in a lifetime. Yet, she never gains a pound. Why?

We are exactly the same height, I have way more muscle than her, but I still had to watch every calorie while she packed away cartloads of food—what the hell was going on here?

If the endocrinologist said she needed some hormone intervention, I'd have proof they were just out for cash.

Long story short, the day her results came in, I got schooled.

"Vanessa, I've read your report, and I'm amazed," the doctor said. "You have the testosterone level of an eighteen-year-old boy. Your growth hormone is perfect. Your thyroid is extremely healthy. You are in flawless shape. Don't do a thing."

Vanessa thanked the doctor and chatted a bit as I sat there, getting more and more pissed off. I love my girl V, but man, how'd she get so lucky?

I was determined to find out how. After working my ass off for so many years, I wanted to be like her.

WHAT DOES "METABOLISM" MEAN, ANYWAY?

Most people throw the word *metabolism* around and feel pretty confident that they know what it means. We say things like "I have a slow metabolism," or "He must have a fast metabolism," about how easily people gain or lose weight. This is an expression of what metabolism does, but it says nothing about what it actually *is*. So what is it? And can it be damaged or enhanced?

We tend to think of metabolism as a furnace, but it's actually more like a chemistry lab. Your metabolism is the combination of all the molecules, hormones, and brain-, gut-, and fat-cell messenger chemicals that regulate the rate at which you burn calories. As you eat, the enzymes in your digestive tract break down the food: proteins turn into amino acids, fats into fatty acids, and carbohydrates into glucose. The blood brings each component to the cells, and their arrival triggers chemical reactions that determine how each is used, or metabolized. Whether this energy will be burned now, stored as fat, or used to build muscle is all in the hands of hormones.

Basically, all metabolic activities can go one of two ways:

Catabolic activities are about destruction—they break apart larger molecules (like the carbohydrates, fats, and protein in our food) to release the fuel that allows the body to function. This process not only gives us the energy to walk around and smile and think but also to build body tissues in anabolic activities.

Anabolic activities are about construction—cells take the glucose, fatty acids, and amino acids from catabolism and turn them into body tissues, like muscles, fat, and bone.

Many hormones that impact our weight are typically put into one of these two categories. For example, cortisol is considered a catabolic hormone; growth hormone is considered an anabolic hormone. Neither catabolic nor anabolic hormones are fully good or bad—you need both kinds of hormones for your metabolism to function normally. The trick is to have the right balance of hormones, like Vanessa, so that you burn fat and build muscle, and not the opposite—nobody wants to build fat and burn muscle.

The differences between Vanessa's hormone test and mine were like night and day. I was really forced to take a look at them and ask myself, "Why? How did this happen?" I started to consider the differences between us:

I had dieted and cut calories for, oh, about fifteen years.
Vanessa had never been on a diet.
I had eaten tons of faux food, fat-free this and low-carb that.
Vanessa ate whole foods—always had.
I drank a six-pack of Diet Coke a day.
Vanessa never drank soda, ever.
I didn't pay attention to where or how my food was grown or produced.
Vanessa ate organic whenever possible.

I kept going through the "I do/she does" list until my head hurt. The results were at times depressing, but ultimately they helped to point the way out of my predicament.

The good news, and what I learned after (a) freaking out and (b) educating myself, is that if metabolism is your biochemistry, then it is dynamic, not static, and can be changed. For the worse, true, but also for better. Just a few small changes in your diet, habits, and lifestyle can have a major impact on your metabolism and your body's natural ability to build fat and burn muscle—and you don't need to be a biochemist to do it.

If you're after immediate results, and you'd rather just take hormones in the form of a pill or a shot every day, you could go to a doctor, get a prescription, and be done with it. But keep in mind that this approach makes your body dependent on external support, and that doesn't come without serious risks. Instead, this program gets at the deeper roots of the problem, optimizing your body's innate hormone levels and resetting your metabolism naturally.

When you give your body the foods it was built to understand, you support your hormones to do what they're meant to do and make your metabolism work for you, not against you. I'm happy to reap the benefits of a strong metabolism now, but for a long time, my hormones were *not* on my side. I had no idea where they were or what they did, let alone

"NORMAL WEIGHT OBESITY"— DO YOU HAVE IT?

Even if you're not officially overweight, you could be overfat—and that excess fat makes you more susceptible to insulin resistance. Recent Mayo Clinic research shows that many normal-weight adults actually have high body fat—greater than 20 percent for men and 30 percent for women—as well as heart and metabolic disturbances. Researchers found this "normal-body-weight obesity" (what I call "skinny fat") in more than half of the patients with a normal BMI. They also tended to have altered blood lipids (high cholesterol), high leptin (a hormone found in fat that is involved in appetite regulation), and higher rates of metabolic syndrome. Body composition is what really counts, not weight.

know how to make them work for me. Let's start there.

HORMONAL SUPPLY AND DEMAND

Your hormones are chemical messengers that control and coordinate activities throughout your entire body. The main goal of your endocrine system is to maintain homeostasis so that the body has enough—but not too much—insulin, cortisol, thyroid, and so on to make the whole operation function well.

When levels of certain hormones go down, or the body thinks it needs more for whatever reason, glands are triggered. The released hormones then travel through the bloodstream to their specific receptors in tissues and organs all over the body. Each hormone fits into its receptor like a key fits into a lock. When they "click," they activate body processes such as hunger, thirst, digestion, muscle building, fat storage, menstruation, sexual desire. You name it, hormones control it. Once the action is completed, homeostasis is restored—however temporarily—and the whole process starts all over.

The problems begin when we get too much or too little of certain hormones in the body. Maybe your gland overproduces the hormone; maybe the receptors on your cells malfunction and don't bond with the hormones as well as they should. Maybe an organ in your body doesn't work right, such as your liver or your kidneys, and the level of hormones circulating in your body gets way too high. Or maybe your endocrine system receives confusing hormonelike signals from toxins in food or the environment, and mistakenly it releases the wrong hormones in response.

When hormonal "storms" like these hit your body, all bets are off.

Some glands get overstimulated and overproduce; some burn out and fail entirely. In today's world, these endocrine problems almost always happen because of factors in our lifestyle and environment.

The "food" we eat now simply doesn't give our hormones what they need to stay balanced. The chemicals and toxins in the environment send signals to our bodies that make them produce more or fewer hormones than normal. These "endocrine disruptors" are substances that act like hormones, tricking the body into reacting (and often overreacting) to their signals, disrupting the normal, healthy functioning of the endocrine system. We'll talk about the most prevalent endocrine disruptors, and how they impact our metabolism, in chapter 3. But for now, know that when your hormones get disrupted, not only is your health in serious jeopardy, important weight-control functions slow down or stop altogether.

That's why we'll get rid of as many of these external endocrine disruptors as possible. Your hormone distribution system will work smoothly again, and your glands and receptors won't go on strike. We'll get your body back to the business of building muscle, burning fat, and staying healthy and happy.

Let's take a few moments to learn about the major hormonal players in your metabolism and what happens when they get all screwy. Once we know a bit more about how our hormones are meant to work, we can fix them.

HORMONES THAT IMPACT METABOLISM

I think we all know why you're here: You want to lose weight. And I want you to as well. So rather than give you the thousand-page treatise on the comprehensive functioning of the endocrine system, let's zero in on those hormones that have the most impact on your body weight. Because it doesn't matter if you're a twenty-five-year-old frustrated diet addict or a fifty-five-year-old who wants to lose his gut, you have the same metabolic hormones. Even if your hormones are at wildly different levels, the principles of the program will work for anyone.

We'll consider the role each hormone plays in metabolic function, hunger, body fat and lean muscle tissue distribution, energy level, and other aspects of general health. We'll talk about what happens when each hormone is at its optimal level, and what type of damage each does when it gets whacked-out. Once we know all that, we'll have a better grasp of the root causes of many metabolic disturbances we'll talk about in chapter 3. When you know what's happening and why, you'll see why the plan can help you fix it.

Throughout the book, we'll also talk about some more recently discovered players on the metabolic and hormonal scene, such as adiponectin, resistin, CCK, neuropeptide Y, and others. But first, let's focus on the major players:

Insulin
Thyroid
Estrogen and progesterone
Testosterone
DHEA and cortisol
Epinephrine and norepinephrine
Human growth hormone
Leptin and ghrelin

METABOLIC HORMONE #1: INSULIN

We heard a lot about insulin in the days of low-carb diets. And for good reason. Problems with insulin are a root cause of some of the most dangerous health conditions, as insulin affects almost every cell in the body. If you can get a grip on your insulin's ups and downs, you'll be a good way toward restoring your body's hormone power.

Where Insulin Comes From: The pancreas. Perched behind your stomach, the pancreas plays a critical role in how the body reacts to food.

How Insulin Impacts Your Metabolism: Insulin's most important function is to lower the concentration of glucose in your blood. Shortly after you eat food, especially highly processed carbohydrates, your meal is broken down into simple sugars and released into the bloodstream. Within minutes, the pancreas pumps out a series of insulin surges. Insulin then ushers those sugars directly into the liver, where they are converted into glycogen for use by the muscles. Insulin also helps turn glucose into fatty acids and ushers them into fat cells, where they can be stored as fuel to be tapped later. Both of these activities lower the concentration of sugar in the blood, which is very important.

While high levels of blood glucose trigger insulin release, low levels suppress it. Maintaining low levels of insulin—one of the primary goals of the diet—allows your body to more easily tap in to your stored fat for fuel.

(Exercise also helps your muscle cells become more sensitive to insulin and more efficient at using glucose for fuel.) When your insulin-release mechanism works the right way, it helps keep your weight in check. But when it's not working, watch out!

How Insulin Gets Out of Whack: Problems arise when your body starts creating too much insulin, which can happen for several reasons. You can probably guess the most common one: when you eat too many of the wrong carbohydrates too often, especially refined carbs like white bread or pasta, which increase your blood sugar dramatically. To cope with this increase, your pancreas delivers a proportionate amount of insulin to scoop it all up into the cells.

For example, let's say you had a Milky Way on an empty stomach. Your blood sugar surge is then so dramatic that insulin overreacts and works twice as hard to clean the sugar out of the blood. This overefficient sugar removal doesn't leave enough glucose circulating in your bloodstream, so your blood sugar concentration drops, you feel hungry again, and you crave (and probably eat) more carbs. That's the postsugar "crash-and-binge" cycle, the root of sugar addiction.

When muscles are still filled up from the last snack, where does the insulin put these extra new calories? Straight into fat. And as long as these large amounts of insulin are still lurking in the bloodstream, your body won't have a chance to tap in to your fat stores for fuel—so you won't burn any fat, either.

If you repeat this cycle enough times, your pancreas will overcompensate and produce more insulin, which your cells will eventually start to ignore. This is called insulin resistance, the precursor of Type 2 diabetes and also common among people with a metabolic syndrome—and excess pounds. Turned away at the door of the muscles, the sugar is left to roam the streets of your blood, aimless and homeless.

GOOD FAT, BAD FAT

The jiggle on your hips and butt, the fatty layer directly beneath your skin, is called subcutaneous fat. This fat is not necessarily bad for you—it's where your metabolically positive hormones leptin and adiponectin come from. A recent study by the Joslin Diabetes Center at Harvard found that subcutaneous fat may even help improve your sensitivity to insulin and protect you from diabetes. However, the fat in your gut—aka visceral fat—surrounds your organs and sets off a hormonal firestorm (and not the good kind). Dr. Scott Isaacs, author of *The Leptin Boost Diet,* calls visceral fat "metabolically evil" because it does everything bad: slows metabolism, lowers growth hormone, raises cortisol, creates insulin resistance, and increases your risk of all kinds of diseases, including diabetes, heart disease, high blood pressure, and fatty liver disease.

If that homeless sugar hangs around the blood too long, doctors call this impaired fasting glucose (if measured in the morning) or impaired glucose tolerance (if measured two hours after a meal). If left unchecked, both conditions can eventually lead to full-blown diabetes.

The more body fat you have, the more insulin is in your brain. And just as our bodies can become insulin-resistant, so can our brains. A longitudinal study found that men who had insulin response problems at fifty were more likely to have cognitive decline, vascular dementia, or Alzheimer's thirty-five years later than men who had normal insulin response.

While you may have heard that obesity causes insulin resistance and diabetes—and it does—another plausible sequence is that insulin resistance comes first, spikes insulin production and blood sugar, and *makes people fat*. (We'll talk about some more surprising—and terrifying—sources of the insulin resistance epidemic in chapter 3.)

THINGS THAT MESS UP INSULIN	SIGNS THAT YOU HAVE TOO LITTLE INSULIN	SIGNS THAT YOU HAVE TOO MUCH INSULIN (AND INSULIN RESISTANCE)	CONDITIONS ASSOCIATED WITH MESSED-UP INSULIN
Certain food additives	Blurred vision	Abdominal obesity (more than 40 inches for men and 35 inches for women)	Diabetes
Certain pesticides	Fatigue	Acne	Heart disease
Certain plastics	Increased pulse rate	Dark patches on armpits, neck, groin, or elbows (acanthosis nigricans)	Impaired glucose tolerance
Certain prescription drugs	Increased urination	Depression	Metabolic syndrome
High-glycemic carbs	Infections (such as yeast infections or genital irritation)	Difficulty sleeping	PCOS
Infections	Rapid breathing	Elevated triglycerides	Prediabetes/impaired fasting glucose
Lack of exercise	Stomach pain	Elevated liver enzymes (fatty liver disease)	Kidney disease
Liver or kidney dysfunction	Unusual thirst	Facial hair (on women)	Gallstones

THINGS THAT MESS UP INSULIN	SIGNS THAT YOU HAVE TOO LITTLE INSULIN	SIGNS THAT YOU HAVE TOO MUCH INSULIN (AND INSULIN RESISTANCE)	CONDITIONS ASSOCIATED WITH MESSED-UP INSULIN
Not eating breakfast	Vomiting	Fasting glucose higher than 100 mg/dL	Gestational diabetes/ high iron production (Hemochromatosis)
Obesity	Weight loss	Fatigue	Sleep apnea
Pregnancy		Gout	
Skipping meals		High blood pressure	
Smoking		Infertility	
Steroids (chronic use)		Irregular menstrual cycles	
Stress		Low sex drive	
Too few calories		Lowered "good" cholesterol (HDL)	
Too many calories		Obesity	
		Skin tags	

METABOLIC HORMONE #2: THYROID

Hypothyroidism has become a bit of a hot health topic these days, following Oprah's revelation of having "blown out" her thyroid gland. I can relate—the same thing happened to me. The truth is, thyroid problems are very common in this country. About 27 million people have a thyroid imbalance, but less than half of them know it, because the symptoms—changes in energy, mood, weight—are similar to many other conditions.

Where Thyroid Hormones Come From: Your thyroid gland, a butterfly-shaped gland located in your neck just below your Adam's apple and just above your collarbone. Normally, it's pretty small—only about two inches, with a lobe on each side of the windpipe. But if your thyroid gets inflamed, you could develop a goiter, where you can actually see a bulge appear on your throat.

How Thyroid Hormones Affect Metabolism: Thyroid hormones perform a ton of functions in your body: They help control the amount of oxygen each cell uses, the rate at which your body burns calories, your heart rate, overall growth, body temperature, fertility, digestion, and your memory and mood. (Basically, the whole enchilada.)

Your pituitary gland creates thyroid-stimulating hormone (TSH) to kick-start the thyroid. The thyroid then grabs iodine out of your blood and turns it into thyroid hormones. The largest amount is T4, thyroxine, which is actually kind of a metabolic dud. The thyroid magic happens when T4 is converted to T3, the zippy metabolism-boosting thyroid hormone. This conversion is fickle and completely dependent upon what's going on in your body. Whether you're sick, stressed, eating well or poorly, pregnant, on medication, getting older, absorbing environmental toxins—all of this will impact how efficiently this conversion happens and, consequently, how much active T3 your body has at any given moment. For example, when you're not taking in enough calories, the pituitary gland stops producing enough TSH, and the thyroid doesn't produce enough T4. Less T4, less T3. Less T3, slower metabolism. This is part of what creates the vicious cycle known as yo-yo dieting.

How Thyroid Hormones Get Out of Whack: When thyroid hormones get unbalanced, either too high or too low, chemical reactions all over the body get thrown off. An underactive thyroid can lower your energy and make you gain weight. Called hypothyroidism, you can feel sluggish and start to pile on extra pounds that you can't blame on a poor diet or lack of exercise. (See "Mastering Hypothyroid" on page 219.)

Most of my clients who are hypothyroid tend to be about fifteen pounds overweight. Same with me. Since I started my thyroid medication—and this diet—I'm back down to my fighting weight and I maintain it with moderate effort. I still exercise and I don't overeat, but I am not killing myself in the gym or starving my body either.

The most common cause of hypothyroidism is Hashimoto's thyroiditis, a hereditary condition seven times more common in women than in men in which the immune system attacks the thyroid. So you can see that women are royally screwed in the thyroid department. All the more reason to get your thyroid tested if you suspect you have one or more of the symptoms listed here. The good news is that this diet will help support your thyroid so it can get to work burning some fat for you.

Given that hypothyroidism can make everything slow down, you might think that being hyperthyroid would be a good thing, right? Not so much. In Graves' disease, the most common form of hyperthyroidism, your heart can race, you can become intolerant to warmer temperatures, and you can lose weight and/or get very tired. People with overactive thyroid glands are sometimes given radioactive iodine, which then makes them *hypo*thyroid. So you can see that thyroid balance is really tricky, with unpleasant effects at both ends of the spectrum. That's why it's important to work with a good endocrinologist to keep your levels well balanced.

THINGS THAT CAN MESS UP THYROID HORMONES	SIGNS THAT YOU HAVE TOO LITTLE THYROID HORMONES	SIGNS THAT YOU HAVE TOO MUCH THYROID HORMONES	CONDITIONS ASSOCIATED WITH MESSED-UP THYROID HORMONES
Certain foods, especially excess iodine	"Brain fog"	Diarrhea	Graves' disease
Environmental toxins	Carpal tunnel syndrome	Dizziness	Postpartum thyroid dysfunction
Extreme dieting	Coarse hair and skin	Emotional instability	Thyroiditis
Genetics	Confusion and forgetfulness	Excessive body heat	
Medicines (lithium and amiodorone)	Constipation	Extreme hunger	
Menopause	Depression	Fast pulse	
Pregnancy	Difficulty swallowing	Fatigue	
Stress	Droopy eyelids	Heat intolerance	
Vitamin deficiencies	Dry and/or yellowing skin	Hyperactivity	
	Exhaustion	Increased hair growth	
	Heavy, prolonged periods	Insomnia	
	High blood pressure	Irritability	
	Hoarse or slow speech	Light or skipped periods	
	Intolerance of cold	Low blood pressure	
	Lethargy/loss of ambition/malaise	Lump on neck	
	Loss of hair	Nervousness	
	Loss of outer third of eyebrow hair	Pounding heartbeat	
	Lump on neck	Prominent eyes ("bug eyes")	
	Muscle cramps, stiffness, and pain	Smooth, moist skin	
	Slow pulse	Sweating	
	Snoring	Weight loss	
	Weight gain/puffy face		

METABOLIC HORMONES #3 AND #4: ESTROGEN AND PROGESTERONE

Estrogen performs an incredible number of roles, especially in women's bodies. In addition to directing a woman's entire development, from child into adult, estrogen also has a major impact on blood fats, digestive enzymes, water and salt balance, bone density, heart function, and memory, among many other functions.

Estrogen and progesterone are steroid hormones. Most people think of muscle-bound meatheads when they hear the word *steroid,* but all it means is that your body creates those hormones out of cholesterol. Men and women both produce estrogen and progesterone normally, but our environment also thrusts a tremendous amount of estrogen on our bodies. Xenoestrogens are man-made estrogens, such as pharmaceutical hormone replacement therapy, environmental toxins (pesticides, plastics, dioxins), and food additives, all of which can have a profound effect on the body's overall estrogen balance. Phytoestrogens are plant sources of estrogen, such as soy and flaxseed, which have a milder effect on the body.

Where Estrogen and Progesterone Are Produced in Women: Ovaries, adrenals, fat tissue, and placenta. Estrogens are actually created throughout the body. They can either bind with receptors on the outside of cells, like other hormones, or scoot directly to receptors in the nucleus, where the DNA lives. These dual powers are part of what makes estrogen so influential.

Women actually have many different kinds of estrogen, but the three main forms are estradiol, estrone, and estriol. Before she hits menopause, the highest amount of naturally produced estrogen in a woman's body is the estradiol from her ovaries, which gets delivered through the entire body within seconds of being created. Estradiol gives women breasts and hips, smooths our skin, protects our brain, heart, and bones, and regulates our menstrual cycle.

Estrone is an estrogen that's produced in our fat cells and our adrenal glands, the walnut-sized glands located right above the kidneys, and has fewer positive things to do in our body. Luckily, before we hit menopause, estrone is easily converted into estradiol. (Afterward, no dice—it stays estrone.)

The third most common estrogen, estriol, isn't nearly as prevalent as the first two. The placenta produces estriol during pregnancy.

Estrogen's buddy, progesterone, comes from the ovaries, where it's released when the follicle bursts and releases your egg every month. Progesterone plays a big part in protecting pregnancy and promoting breast-feeding. Progesterone is also produced in the adrenals, and serves as a precursor to cortisol, testosterone, and estrogen.

Where Estrogen and Progesterone Are Produced in Men: The testes and adrenals. Men have a small amount of natural estradiol, produced in the testes and adrenals. When estrogen is at a normal level, it can help protect a man's brain, heart, and bones as well as maintain a healthy libido.

How Estrogen and Progesterone Impact Women's Metabolism: Estradiol is the estrogen of youth; in proper levels, it primarily helps women's bodies stay lean. Estradiol lowers insulin and blood pressure levels, raises HDL, and lowers LDL. Women with more estradiol tend to have higher levels of muscle and lower levels of fat. Estradiol helps regulate hunger by creating the same satisfied feeling that comes from serotonin. Similarly, it helps keep your moods stable and your energy high, so you're more motivated to exercise. Estradiol does put fat on your hips and butt, but remember—that fat actually helps your insulin response.

As you prepare to go through menopause, your ovaries start to shut down and your production of estradiol decreases. Then estrone becomes your main estrogen, which really sucks. Estrone immediately shifts fat from your butt and hips to your belly. As you lose more of your ovarian estrogen, your body becomes desperate to hang on to other estrogen-making areas of the body, including fat, making it harder for you to lose that belly fat. And the more fat you have, the more estrone you'll produce, because fat tissue turns fat-burning androgens into fat-storing estrone.

Most women tend to gain several pounds during this transition, ramping up what becomes a vicious cycle: more estrone, more fat on the belly; more fat on the belly, more estrone.

Another of estrogen's vicious cycles has to do with insulin. Insulin increases circulating levels of estrogen, and estrone causes insulin resistance. According to the Mayo Clinic, estrogen is fifty to one hundred times higher in postmenopausal women who are overweight than in those who are thinner, which may account for the 20 percent greater risk of cancer (especially breast cancer) among heavier older women.

Progesterone helps to balance estrogen and can help manage some of these issues, so when progesterone levels drop, that creates problems, too. For example, when progesterone drops right before your period, that imbalance may be what triggers cravings to eat, primarily carbs. Progesterone also drops at menopause, even more dramatically than estrogen. Because progesterone is also the precursor for testosterone and estradiol, when your progesterone production falls off, you also start to lose the fat-burning effects of those metabolically positive hormones.

How Estrogen and Progesterone Impact Men's Metabolism: When estrogen is in balance with men's testosterone, it has little negative impact on metabolism. But when estrogen is out of balance with other hormones, men can lose their muscle-building, fat-burning advantage. That's when they tend to develop man-boobs (affectionately known as "moobs") and love handles, features typically seen on women.

How Estrogen and Progesterone Get Out of Whack: People used to think that all of women's hormone balance problems stemmed from declining levels of estrogen, especially during perimenopause and menopause, PMS, or postpartum periods. But increasingly, women in Western cultures tend to have *too much* estrogen rather than too little.

For the past fifty years, doctors have started to notice that girls' puberty changes—budding breasts, pubic hair development, and early menstruation—have been happening earlier and earlier. Rates of breast cancer have jumped 40 percent in the past thirty-five years. And many signs—including decreasing sperm counts and increasing prostate cancer rates—indicate that men are facing the same issue of excessive estrogen.

A large part of this hormonal disruption comes from the overwhelming explosion of xenoestrogens in the environment. We will get into this problem in much greater detail throughout the book, as it is one of the most troubling repercussions of our country's addiction to toxic chemicals. Our bodies are getting slammed with endocrine-disrupting synthetic estrogens, from the ingredients in our cosmetics and the cleansers under our sinks to the preservatives in our foods and the plastics wrapping them. You'll see how the scope of the impact on our hormonal balance is *staggering*.

Other factors can also increase unhealthy levels of estrogen, such as stress, a lack of quality fats or protein, and too many refined grains, sugars, and processed foods. We'll talk about all of these factors, because estrogen overload is one of the most critical crises in our biochemistry today.

Men are naturally prone to increases in estrogen as they age, but any additional excess can lead to further problems with decreased metabolism, muscle building, and libido. For younger men, rising levels of estrogens are almost always a product of environmental estrogens. These excess estrogens put all of us at higher risk of cancer, infertility, diabetes, and other serious conditions.

In contrast with traditional thinking, some researchers now believe that most perimenopausal or menopausal hormonal symptoms are caused not by a dip in estrogen but by a plummet in progesterone. Some believe that too much estrogen and too little progesterone creates "estrogen dominance," a condition that was named by John R. Lee, M.D., one of the first prominent doctors to supplement with bioidentical progesterone to help his patients manage menopause. Dr. Lee's theory is still controversial, but as the evidence of the destructive forces of environmental estrogens piles up, belief in an emerging epidemic of estrogen dominance continues to grow.

Stress can also make this imbalance worse. Cortisol and progesterone compete for the same receptors on your cells, so when you overproduce cortisol, you threaten your healthy progesterone activity. The Master Your Metabolism plan will help you correct your estrogen/progesterone balance by addressing many of these issues. You'll start by identifying and Removing as many exogenous estrogens from your diet and your environment as possible. You'll also Restore the whole foods, especially healthful fats, that help your body build the right hormones, while you Rebalance the stress that can hamper proper hormone production.

THINGS THAT CAN MESS UP ESTROGEN AND PROGESTERONE	SIGNS THAT WOMEN HAVE IMBALANCED ESTROGEN AND PROGESTERONE	SIGNS THAT MEN HAVE IMBALANCED ESTROGEN	CONDITIONS ASSOCIATED WITH MESSED-UP ESTROGEN AND PROGESTERONE
Age	Acid reflux	Breasts	Breast, ovarian, testicular, or adrenal cancer
Birth control pills	Anxiety	Decreased libido	Cirrhosis
Body fat	Belly fat	Decreased muscle tone	Early puberty
Pesticides	Bloating	Depression	Endometriosis
Plastics	"Brain fog"	Enlarged prostate	Fibrocystic breasts
Pollution	Breast buds before age 7	Erectile dysfunction	Hypogonadism
Smoking	Breast cysts	Increased belly fat	Hypopituitarism
Stress	Carb cravings	Increased body fat	Infertility
	Chronic fatigue	Low sperm count	Menopause
	Decreased libido	Low sperm motility	Perimenopause
	Depression	Reduced facial hair	PCOS (polycystic ovarian syndrome)
	Dizziness		PMS
	Dry skin		Uterine fibroids
	Excess facial hair		
	Extreme PMS or premenstrual dysphonic disorder (PMDD)		
	Fatigue		
	Hair loss		
	Heavier or skipped periods		

THINGS THAT CAN MESS UP ESTROGEN AND PROGESTERONE	SIGNS THAT WOMEN HAVE IMBALANCED ESTROGEN AND PROGESTERONE	SIGNS THAT MEN HAVE IMBALANCED ESTROGEN	CONDITIONS ASSOCIATED WITH MESSED-UP ESTROGEN AND PROGESTERONE
	High blood sugar		
	Hot flashes		
	Impaired memory		
	Incontinence		
	Increased asthma or allergies		
	Insomnia		
	Insulin resistance		
	Irritability		
	Irritable bowel syndrome		
	Joint stiffness		
	Migraines		
	Mood swings		
	Night sweats		
	Restless sleep		
	Weight gain		

METABOLIC HORMONES #5 AND #6: TESTOSTERONE AND DHEA

The androgens testosterone and DHEA are not just for guys. Don't worry, ladies—boosting these hormones won't turn us into knuckle-dragging Neanderthals. In fact, they can help increase our energy, make us want to hit the gym, and help us build more calorie-burning muscle. That's why we have to do everything we can to protect their levels, because as we get older, they start to head south.

Where Testosterone and DHEA Come From: The testes, ovaries, and adrenals. Men produce most of their testosterone in their reproductive glands, the testes. Just as estradiol does for women, testosterone helps develop men's secondary sex characteristics, such as body and facial hair. But testosterone helps both guys *and* girls—it boosts libido, keeps energy high, protects bone, and preserves mental function in later years.

Most of women's testosterone comes from their adrenals, which is also the source of their DHEA. A precursor to testosterone (and estradiol), DHEA may help prevent breast cancer, cardiovascular disease, impaired memory and brain function, as well as osteoporosis. Awesome hormone that it is, DHEA may even help us live longer.

How Testosterone and DHEA Impact Your Metabolism: Androgens are, by definition, anabolic hormones—they build rather than destroy. And what they build, thank goodness, is mostly muscle. In both men and women, testosterone helps increase lean muscle mass and strength, boosts libido, and improves energy. In women, testosterone can also be converted to estrogen. Testosterone and DHEA are forces of good in the metabolic war.

How Testosterone and DHEA Get Out of Whack: Testosterone and DHEA are both hormones of youth. As men and women get older, our production of them starts to trend downward. According to Scott Isaacs, about one-third of all women experience low androgen levels at some point in their lives. Starting as early as thirty, men's testosterone dips about 1 to 2 percent per year. In most men, this slow and steady decline of "andropause" is different from women's more rapid loss of estrogen and progesterone (which basically fall off a cliff at menopause). DHEA also declines, and because it's the building block of so many important hormones, all hormone levels suffer.

As we lose these powerful androgens to advancing age, certain things happen: Our libidos slip, our muscles lose mass, we gain abdominal fat, and our bones weaken. Motivation to exercise decreases, which is absolutely tragic because exercise helps to boost testosterone. Men with abnormally low free testosterone levels are almost three times more likely to be depressed than men with high testosterone.

To make matters worse, as people gain weight, their bodies start to convert more of their testosterone to estrogen. This estrogen can then start to overshadow the effects of the testosterone in another vicious cycle: more estrogen, more fat; more fat, more estrogen. The testosterone keeps getting crowded out of the equation.

Testosterone supplementation is a new field for men and women, and although some of the research seems very promising, doctors remain a bit cautious until longer-term studies are completed. One area that's clearly dangerous is when younger people try to supplement their androgens without the help of an endocrinologist. When young men and women take artificial anabolic steroids, they actually train their glands to produce *less* of their own androgens. That's why guys who take 'roids tend to have tiny testicles and high voices—their bodies think they have plenty of male hormones, so they stop producing any of their own. (Kind of the opposite of what they want, right?)

Another risk comes when people self-diagnose "adrenal fatigue"—a very trendy term these high-stress days—and start to supplement with DHEA without consulting an endocrinologist. When done incorrectly, this type of supplementation can do one of two things:

- Hamper adrenal hormone production (because your adrenals now believe you have enough circulating hormones and stop making their own)
- Cause your body to convert the excess DHEA into excess estrogen (which can worsen your problems with body fat and exacerbate cancer risks)

Bottom line: Don't mess around with supplementation without medical assistance. You're much better off optimizing your body's natural production of androgens. You can do that by protecting your adrenals—the source of more than 50 percent of women's androgen production—and making sure you have plenty of good-quality fats and protein, as well as vitamins and minerals (like B vitamins and zinc) to build these critical steroids.

On the other end of the spectrum, some women develop PCOS, a syndrome in which they have too much androgen. (See "Mastering PCOS" on page 224.) PCOS is intricately related to insulin resistance, but researchers are still not 100 percent sure of what causes it. Women with PCOS often have irregular periods, abnormal hair growth, and trouble getting pregnant. Unfortunately, the excess androgens and insulin resistance also send a lot of fat directly to women's bellies, mimicking male-pattern weight gain. Because we still don't know exactly where it comes from, our best chance of avoiding PCOS is to manage our insulin levels—which is job number one on this diet.

THINGS THAT MESS UP TESTOSTERONE AND/OR DHEA	SIGNS THAT YOU HAVE TOO LITTLE TESTOSTERONE AND/OR DHEA	SIGNS THAT YOU HAVE TOO MUCH TESTOSTERONE AND/OR DHEA	SOME CONDITIONS ASSOCIATED WITH MESSED-UP TESTOSTERONE AND/OR DHEA
Aging	Anxiety	Acne	Andropause (male menopause)

continued on the following page

(continued)

THINGS THAT MESS UP TESTOSTERONE AND/OR DHEA	SIGNS THAT YOU HAVE TOO LITTLE TESTOSTERONE AND/OR DHEA	SIGNS THAT YOU HAVE TOO MUCH TESTOSTERONE AND/OR DHEA	SOME CONDITIONS ASSOCIATED WITH MESSED-UP TESTOSTERONE AND/OR DHEA
Body fat	Beer belly	Aggression	Infertility
Diabetes	Changes in body composition	Balding	Polycystic ovarian syndrome
Insulin resistance	Decreased libido	Excessive body hair growth	
Lack of exercise	Depression	High blood pressure	
Pituitary tumor	Erectile dysfunction	Irregular periods	
Stress	Fatigue	Lowered voice	
Taking steroids	Lack of motivation	Overactive sex drive	
Too little progesterone	Loss of muscle mass		
Too much estrogen	Man-boobs		
Trauma to the testes	Reduced bone density		
	Smaller testes		
	Thicker waist		

METABOLIC HORMONES #7, #8, AND #9: NOREPINEPHRINE, EPINEPHRINE, AND CORTISOL

Our fight-or-flight hormones can get us out of some pretty tight squeezes. They help us make deadlines, save toddlers from tripping down stairs, and run to catch buses. But while the effects of heart-pumping epinephrine and norepinephrine are fleeting, fat-storing cortisol's legacy is longer lasting—and deadly.

Where Norepinephrine, Epinephrine, and Cortisol Are Produced: The adrenal glands. Cortisol, also called hydrocortisone, is produced in the adrenal cortex, the outer part of each adrenal gland. The inner part of the adrenal gland, the adrenal medulla, produces the other primary stress hormones, norepinephrine (which restricts blood vessels, increasing blood pressure) and epinephrine (which increases heart rate and blood flow to muscles). Each of these stress hormones is released in different ratios based on the challenge you face. If you're looking at a challenge that you think you can handle, your adrenals release more norepinephrine. (And after you win, you release more testosterone as you savor the victory.) If you face a challenge that seems more difficult, something you're not sure you can master, you release more epinephrine, the "anxiety hormone." But when you're overwhelmed, totally discouraged, and convinced you're screwed, you release more cortisol. That distinction has led some researchers to call cortisol "the hormone of defeat."

How Norepinephrine, Epinephrine, and Cortisol Impact Metabolism: When you first become stressed, norepinephrine will tell your body to stop producing insulin so that you can have plenty of fast-acting blood glucose ready. Similarly, epinephrine will relax the muscles of the stomach and intestines and decrease blood flow to these organs. (Your body figures it would rather focus on saving your life than digesting your food.) These two actions cause some of the high blood sugar and stomach problems associated with stress.

Once the stressor has passed, cortisol tells the body to stop producing these hormones and to resume digestion. But cortisol continues to have a huge impact on your blood sugar, particularly on how your body uses fuel. A catabolic hormone, cortisol tells your body what fat, protein, or carbohydrates to burn and when to burn them, depending on what kind of challenge you face. Cortisol can either take your fat, in the form of triglycerides, and move it to your muscle, or break down muscle and convert it into glycogen for more energy. (That's not all it breaks down. Excess cortisol also deconstructs bone and skin, leading to osteoporosis, easy bruising, and—ugh—stretch marks.)

While the epinephrine (aka adrenaline) rush of acute stress suppresses appetite—who really wants to eat when a bully is about to punch you?—any cortisol hanging around after the fact will stimulate it. If you haven't released the excess cortisol in your blood by punching back or running away, cortisol will increase your cravings for high-fat, high-carb foods. Cortisol also lowers leptin levels and increases levels of neuropeptide Y (NPY), shifts proven to stimulate appetite.

Once you eat, your body releases a cascade of rewarding brain chemicals that can set up an addictive relationship with food. You feel stressed, you eat. Your body releases natural opioids, you feel better. If you don't consciously avoid this pattern, you can become physically and psychologically dependent on that release to manage stress. It's no coincidence that stress eaters who self-medicate with food tend to have hair-trigger epinephrine reactions and chronically high levels of cortisol.

When stress continues for a long time, and cortisol levels remain high, the body actually resists weight loss. Your body thinks times are hard and you might starve, so it greedily hoards any food you eat and any fat already present on your body. Cortisol also turns adipocytes, young fat cells, into mature fat cells that stick with us forever.

Cortisol tends to take fat from healthier areas, like your butt and hips, and move it to your abdomen, where cortisol has more receptors. In the process, it turns once-healthy peripheral fat into unhealthy visceral fat that increases inflammation and insulin resistance in the body. This belly fat then leads to more cortisol because it has higher concentrations of a specific enzyme that converts inactive cortisone to active cortisol. The more belly fat you have, the more active cortisol will be converted by these enzymes—yet another vicious cycle created by visceral fat.

How Norepinephrine, Epinephrine, and Cortisol Get Out of Whack: Depending on genes and early childhood experiences, some lucky people may have very mellow adrenal reactions to stressful situations. Many other people, however, tend to overrespond, even to minor threats, because the stress feedback loop became stronger and stronger with each negative experience in their past. By the time these people are adults, their bodies have very touchy stress-response systems.

Chronic overstimulation of our adrenals is epidemic in this country. We are both victims of and addicted to our stress. And our bodies pay the price. Long-term activation of the stress system has a lethal effect on the body. When you abuse your adrenals as much as we do, you set yourself up for heart disease, diabetes, stroke, and other potentially fatal conditions. But before you even get there, you could completely fry your adrenals.

"Adrenal fatigue" is a trendy term tossed around quite a bit right now. Mainstream medicine has not officially recognized the syndrome (supposedly characterized by insomnia, weight gain, depression, acne, hair loss, carb cravings, and lowered immune function), but some endocrinologists have built their practices on helping patients reverse these symptoms.

If you suspect either abnormally high or abnormally low cortisol levels, this plan is the perfect way to give your body the best nutrition and lifestyle strategies to support yourself in times of stress. When you limit your caffeine to 200 milligrams a day, avoid simple carbs, processed foods, and refined grains, and get plenty of high-quality protein, in addition to following the de-stressing strategies I'll share with you in chapter 8, you'll automatically help your body keep your stress hormones, especially cortisol, lower.

If you still need some help, work with a credentialed endocrinologist to assess your levels before doing any kind of supplementation. **Please do not take any over-the-counter "adrenal support" supplements— you could actually push your body into full-blown adrenal insufficiency, a very serious, potentially fatal condition.**

THINGS THAT CAN MESS UP CORTISOL LEVELS	SIGNS THAT YOU HAVE TOO LITTLE CORTISOL	SIGNS THAT YOU HAVE TOO MUCH CORTISOL	SOME CONDITIONS ASSOCIATED WITH MESSED-UP CORTISOL
Aggression	Changes in blood pressure or heart rate	Belly fat	Addison's disease
Anger	Chronic diarrhea	Depression	Adrenal insufficiency
Conflict	Darkening of the skin or patchy skin color	Diabetes	Cushing's syndrome
Depression	Extreme weakness	Easily bruised skin	Diabetes
Diabetes	Fatigue	Frequent infections or colds	Hirsutism
Dieting	Lesions inside the mouth	High blood pressure	Hypoglycemia
Excessive caffeine	Loss of appetite	High blood sugar	Insulin resistance
Excessive sugar	Low blood pressure	High cholesterol and triglycerides	
Fear	Nausea and vomiting	Insomnia	
Infrequent meals	Paleness	Insulin resistance	
Lack of sleep	Salt craving	Irregular periods	
Over-the-counter "adrenal support" supplements	Slow, sluggish movements	Obesity	
Prolonged stress	Unnaturally dark skin color in some places	Reduced libido	
Skipping breakfast	Unintentional weight loss	Weight gain	
Unhealthy psychological habits			

METABOLIC HORMONE #10: GROWTH HORMONE

Growth hormone (sometimes called HGH) is one of those hormones that we all want more of. It seems to make everything better—it builds muscle, burns fat, helps you resist heart disease, protects your bones, increases your overall health, and some say it even makes you happier. People with higher levels of growth hormone live longer, and better. But don't get HGH shots just yet—supplementation is controversial and risky, and may even cause insulin resistance. One of the primary goals of this program is to protect and increase your natural production of growth hormone.

Where Growth Hormone Is Produced: The pituitary, a tiny gland nestled underneath the hypothalamus in the brain. Growth hormone is one of the most influential anabolic hormones, playing a huge role in the growth of bone and other body tissue while also enhancing immunity.

How Growth Hormone Impacts Metabolism: Growth hormone increases your muscle mass in several ways: It helps your body absorb amino acids, helps synthesize them into muscle, and then prevents the muscle from breaking down. All these actions raise your resting metabolic rate and give you more power for your workouts.

Growth hormone is also amazing at helping you tap in to your fat stores. Fat cells have growth hormone receptors that trigger your cells to break down and burn your triglycerides. Growth hormone also discourages your fat cells from absorbing or holding on to any fat floating around in your bloodstream.

Add to these amazing feats the fact that growth hormone can be your liver's best friend. It helps to maintain and protect the pancreatic islets that produce insulin and also helps the liver synthesize glucose. Growth hormone promotes gluconeogenesis, a really cool process by which the body can create carbs out of protein. Gluconeogenesis helps you lose fat faster while providing your brain and other tissues with the energy they need, without excess dietary carbs.

Growth hormone actually counters insulin's ability to shuttle glucose into cells, nudging it into the liver instead. Unfortunately, this action is one of the reasons excess supplemental growth hormone can cause insulin resistance—which is why you have to be very careful before you go down that road.

How Growth Hormone Gets Out of Whack: Growth hormone deficiency is a very real condition, especially detrimental in childhood. Kids without enough growth hormone end up shorter and have delayed sexual development, and their growth hormone shortfall can continue into adulthood. Growth hormone deficiency can begin in adulthood as well, but can be harder to diagnose then, as symptoms include some common characteristics of aging, such as declining bone mass, energy, and strength.

The fact that this medically definable condition exists has given some antiaging clinics the latitude to supplement their patients interested in growth hormone's fat-burning, muscle-building traits. Just as in menopause and andropause, the sad fact is that growth hormone naturally starts to decline sometime after our thirties. But we also do many things that hasten that decline prematurely, and we should look to change those behaviors before we ever consider supplementation.

Of all the less-than-smart things we do to mess up our hormone balance, depriving ourselves of good-quality sleep is probably the dumbest. Growth hormone is released in adults in an average of five pulses throughout each day. The largest of these pulses happens during our deepest, stage 4 sleep, about one hour after we first drop off. A University of Chicago study found that when people are deprived of this stage of sleep (with minor disturbances that didn't quite wake them but interfered with the quality of their sleep), their daily growth hormone levels fell 23 percent.

Another way we surpress our own growth hormone levels is when we eat too many low-quality carbs and keep our blood sugar and insulin high. Protein, on the other hand, can help release higher levels of growth hormone, so if we shortchange ourselves there, in favor of carbs, we slam our production on two levels. New evidence is also starting to emerge that hormones from pesticides and other contaminants in our environment and diet can impact our growth hormone levels.

One surefire way we turn our bodies into growth hormone factories is with intense exercise. During intense exercise, and especially during intervals, growth hormone shuns glucose and instead encourages the body to use fat as its fuel. Not only does this help you burn fat while you exercise, it keeps your blood glucose level stable so that you have the energy to keep exercising. When you don't exercise and your muscles become insulin-resistant, you increase your level of circulating insulin, and you suppress growth hormone even further. We need to get off our butts and capitalize on this incredibly healthy way to reverse aging—not jab ourselves with HGH syringes!

The Master Your Metabolism diet incorporates all of the proven ways to naturally boost growth hormone: stress relief, rest, and improved sleep; balanced blood sugar and high-quality protein; and just enough intense exercise to burn fat, improve insulin sensitivity, and flush toxins from the body.

THINGS THAT CAN MESS UP GROWTH HORMONE	SIGNS THAT YOU HAVE TOO LITTLE GROWTH HORMONE	SIGNS THAT YOU HAVE TOO MUCH GROWTH HORMONE	CONDITIONS ASSOCIATED WITH MESSED-UP GROWTH HORMONE
Environmental toxins	Decreased bone density	Carpal tunnel syndrome	Growth hormone deficiency
Excess estrogens	Decreased exercise performance	Diabetes	
High blood sugar	Decreased libido	Hardening of the arteries	
High cortisol	Decreased muscle mass	High blood pressure	
Late nights (up until midnight or later)	Decreased muscle strength	Insulin resistance	
Nonorganic meats and dairy	Depression or mood swings	Male breast enlargement (man-boobs)	
Not enough exercise	Fatty deposits in face and belly	Sexual dysfunction	
Not enough total hours of sleep	Higher levels of insulin	Thickening of bones in jaw, fingers, and toes	
Shallow sleep (no slow-wave stage 3 or 4 sleep)	Lowered energy level		
Stress	Short stature		
Too much dietary fat	Sleep problems		
	Unhealthy levels of LDL		
	Wrinkles		

METABOLIC HORMONE #11: LEPTIN

Scientists used to believe that fat cells were just big blobs of yuck waiting to get bigger or smaller. Now they know that our fat is an enormous endocrine gland, actively producing and reacting to hormones. While scientists continue to identify more and more fat cell hormones every day, perhaps the best studied of these hormones is leptin.

Where Leptin Is Produced: Fat cells. Leptin is a protein, made by fat cells, that is controlled by an influential gene called the ob gene. Leptin works with other hormones—thyroid, cortisol, and insulin—to help your body figure out how hungry it is, how fast it will burn off the food you eat, and if it will hang on to (or let go of) weight.

How Leptin Impacts Your Metabolism: You have receptors for leptin scattered everywhere, but your brain is where this hormone is most active. When you've eaten a meal, the fat cells throughout your body release this hormone. Leptin travels to the hypothalamus, the part of the brain that helps regulate appetite, and bonds with leptin receptors there. These receptors control the production of neuropeptides, small signaling proteins that switch our appetites on and off.

One of the most well known of these is neuropeptide Y, the peptide that turns on the appetite and turns down the metabolic rate. Leptin switches off neuropeptide Y, switches on appetite-suppressing signals, and the body gets the message to stop being hungry and start burning more calories.

When it's working the right way, leptin also helps the body tap in to longer-term fat stores and reduce them. But when leptin signaling doesn't work, you keep eating because you never feel like you've had enough food.

In addition to the leptin release you get after eating, your body also experiences a leptin surge overnight, while you sleep. This leptin surge boosts your levels of thyroid-stimulating hormone, which helps the thyroid release thyroxine.

How Leptin Gets Out of Whack: Leptin can go wrong in several ways. One, you could be born with low levels of leptin. Scientists have found that a mutation of the *ob* gene hurts our leptin production; this mutation causes certain children to become severely obese. Simple supplementation with leptin usually helps these children maintain a healthy weight. This condition is extremely rare—you would *definitely* know by now if you had it.

Believe it or not, low levels are not our biggest leptin problem. Researchers are finding that many people who are overweight actually have very high levels of leptin. How could this be? Well, the more fat you have, the more leptin you produce. And similar to what happens in insulin resistance, when the body continually cranks out excess levels of leptin—in response to overeating—the receptors for leptin can start to get worn out and no longer recognize it. People with leptin resistance have high levels of circulating leptin, but their receptors cannot accept it, neuropeptide Y never gets shut off, they remain hungry, and their metabolism slows down. (This high level of neuropeptide Y also interferes with your T4 activity, further damaging your metabolism.)

Leptin resistance and insulin resistance go hand in hand, but just like with insulin resistance, if you lose a bit of weight, your body will become more sensitive to leptin and it will start acting the way it was intended to—to help you push away from the table and say, "Enough!"

THINGS THAT CAN MESS UP LEPTIN	SIGNS THAT YOU HAVE TOO LITTLE LEPTIN	SIGNS THAT YOU HAVE TOO MUCH LEPTIN (AND YOUR BODY HAS BECOME RESISTANT TO IT)	CONDITIONS ASSOCIATED WITH MESSED-UP LEPTIN
Abdominal fat	Anorexia nervosa	Constant hunger	Diabetes
Aging	Constant hunger	Diabetes	Fatty liver disease
High bad-carb diet	Depression	Elevated thyroid hormones	Gallstones
High trans fat diet		Heart disease	Heart disease
Infections		High blood pressure	High blood lipids (LDL, triglycerides)
Inflammation		Higher cholesterol	High blood pressure
Menopause		Increased inflammation	Insulin resistance
Not enough REM sleep (or less than 7 to 8 hours of continuous sleep)		Obesity	PCOS

THINGS THAT CAN MESS UP LEPTIN	SIGNS THAT YOU HAVE TOO LITTLE LEPTIN	SIGNS THAT YOU HAVE TOO MUCH LEPTIN (AND YOUR BODY HAS BECOME RESISTANT TO IT)	CONDITIONS ASSOCIATED WITH MESSED-UP LEPTIN
Obesity			Skin tags
Pain			Testosterone deficiency
Smoking			
Stress			

▶ METABOLIC HORMONE #12: GHRELIN

Leptin and ghrelin act in kind of a yin-yang balance between hunger and satisfaction. Just as leptin tells the brain to turn off hunger, ghrelin tells the brain that you're famished.

Where Ghrelin Is Produced: The stomach, duodenum, and upper intestine. When you're hungry, about to eat, or even just thinking about eating something delicious, your gut releases ghrelin. Acting as a messenger, ghrelin then travels up to your hypothalamus and turns on neuropeptide Y, which increases your appetite and decreases metabolic burn. Ghrelin has one good thing going for it, though—it helps the pituitary release growth hormone.

How Ghrelin Impacts Your Metabolism: In your average Jane, ghrelin goes up when the stomach is empty. This hormone is the reason you always feel hungry at particular moments in the day—your body's clock triggers the release of ghrelin according to a finely tuned schedule. Ghrelin levels will stay up until you've given your body enough nutrients to satisfy its needs. Because those signals can take a few minutes to kick in, eating slowly may help you to eat less overall. By the time your stomach fills up, ghrelin levels start to drop again, you feel satisfied, and you can stop eating.

Interestingly, it's not ghrelin itself that makes you feel hungry—that hunger is stimulated in part by neuropeptide Y and also by the growth hormone it releases. In fact, ghrelin levels *must* rise to allow the release of growth hormone. That's just one of the many reasons why this plan

A FEW MORE METABOLIC HORMONES

In the past few decades, scientists have discovered dozens of hormones that impact weight, fat stores, hunger, cravings, and metabolism. While we focus on the twelve major hormones in this chapter, the plan works to balance the following hormones and peptides as well.

Adiponectin: Created by the fat throughout your body—mostly in your butt!—adiponectin is a hormonal good guy. It improves the function of your liver and blood vessels, lowering your blood sugar and guarding your body against insulin and leptin resistance. Low levels of adiponectin are associated with inflammation and metabolic syndrome.

Cholecystokinin (CCK): A natural appetite suppressant, neuropeptide CCK is created near the top of your small intestine after you eat a meal—especially one with fiber, fat, or protein—to tell your brain that you're no longer hungry. CCK acts quickly, with a half-life of 1 to 2 minutes, and then resets for the next meal.

Glucagonlike peptide (GLP-1): Also created in the small intestine, especially when you eat carbs and fat, GLP-1 stimulates the pancreas to stop producing glucagon and start producing insulin. GLP-1 also slows down your digestion, keeping your appetite low.

Neuropeptide Y (NPY): NPY is not your friend. Activated by ghrelin, neuropeptide NPY makes you want to eat—a lot—and stimulates your body to store fat. Both extreme dieting and overeating/weight gain tend to increase the activity of NPY. It is created in the brain and in belly fat cells, and it stimulates the birth of new fat cells, too. (Like I said, not your friend.)

Obestatin: Although controlled by the same gene that controls ghrelin, and also produced in the gut, obestatin actually works the opposite of ghrelin—it tells your brain that you're *not* hungry and that you should eat less.

Peptide tyrosine-tyrosine (peptide YY, or PYY): PYY is also released when your belly expands after a meal and also decreases your appetite, primarily by blocking the action of NPY. Fat and protein seem to raise PYY the most, but fasting for two or three days can cut PYY levels by 50 percent. PYY's effects last longer than other gut hormones—it starts to climb within 30 minutes of eating and stays high for up to two hours afterward.

Resistin: This evil hormone plays a big role in insulin resistance, blocking the ability of muscles to respond to insulin. Some experts even think it may be *the* link between obesity and insulin resistance. Your belly fat produces 15 times more resistin than your peripheral fat does—all the more reason to lose that gut!

does not allow eating after nine P.M.—I want that food to be nearly out of your system by the time you head to bed.

Your body requires ghrelin to enable you to move effectively through all the necessary phases of sleep. Without the proper progression, you won't get to stage 4 sleep, during which you get a big pulse of growth hormone, or to the REM sleep that helps protect leptin levels. For the rest of the day, though, the object is to keep ghrelin levels low. You don't need the extra diet-endangering hunger and all the metabolic havoc those resulting blood sugar ups and downs wreak on your system.

THINGS THAT CAN MESS UP GHRELIN	SIGNS THAT YOU HAVE TOO LITTLE GHRELIN	SIGNS THAT YOU HAVE TOO MUCH (OR A HIGHER SENSITIVITY TO) GHRELIN	CONDITIONS ASSOCIATED WITH MESSED-UP GHRELIN
Binge eating	Development of eating disorders	Constant hunger	Anorexia nervosa
Eating too much fat	Disinterest in eating		Binge eating disorder
Less than 8 hours of sleep a night	Weight loss		Bulimia nervosa
Low thyroid levels			Prader-Willi Syndrome
Not eating enough protein or carbs			
Severe dieting			
Skipping meals			
Stress			

How Ghrelin Gets Out of Whack: You have to stay ahead of those ghrelin surges, because ghrelin is crafty about getting you to eat. New research shows that it triggers reward centers in the brain to make food look more appetizing. These areas of the brain have been linked to drug addiction for many years, and researchers believe ghrelin triggers these centers even when you don't have any reason to eat—other than passing a bakery just as the bread comes out of the oven.

Constant calorie restriction keeps ghrelin levels high, which may be why some yo-yo dieters feel like their hunger just keeps getting worse the fewer calories they eat. This is all part of nature's way of getting us to eat, eat already. As we walk around in a world of way too much French bread, this ever-rising ghrelin is probably a big part of what makes maintaining weight loss so challenging.

Interestingly, a select group of people may feel better when they have higher levels of ghrelin. People with anorexia nervosa actually have much higher levels of ghrelin than average people, whereas people with binge-eating disorder have lower levels. Binge eaters' ghrelin production may take a hit after they repeatedly eat well beyond the point where ghrelin is no longer making them hungry—as with other hormones, their hormonal feedback system no longer works. On the other hand, animal studies suggest that increases in ghrelin may help some people manage depression caused by chronic stress. Perhaps in people with anorexia, ghrelin acts almost as an antidepressant.

A reduction in ghrelin levels might even be one of the ways that gastric bypass surgery reduces people's weight. When you go into your stomach and literally remove the cells that produce ghrelin, you feel less hunger. But I don't know—this seems a tad extreme to me. We can come up with better ways to manage your ghrelin than going under the knife—like eating balanced meals every four hours and hitting the sheets for eight hours a night. That doesn't sound so bad, does it?

▶ PREPARE TO BE SCARED

Every choice you make in your life impacts this very complex chemistry: where you live, how long you sleep, whether or not you have kids, what you do (or don't do) for exercise, who's dumping what into your water supply. Now, we can't change everything, but we do have a great deal of power over what we put in our mouths, on our skin, and in our minds.

First, let's take a look at what's causing all these problems. Be prepared to get scared. When I first found out, I certainly was. Once you know what you're up against, you'll learn how to restore your metabolism and put your fat-burning hormones to work again.

CHAPTER 3

HOW YOU GOT THIS WAY

WHY THE LAND OF PLENTY IS NOT GOOD—
IN MORE WAYS THAN ONE

I bet you know at least one person who can eat everything in sight and still struggle to keep the weight *on*. The woman who lost sixty pregnancy pounds in a month. The guy who puts away three burgers at a sitting but still wears the same jeans he wore in high school.

I don't know about you, but I can't do that. My metabolism will not allow it. So where did my slowpoke metabolism come from and how do I change it? Can I please just blame my parents and be done with it? Isn't it all in the genes?

Not so fast. Genes are only a slice of the picture—some scientists estimate that genes are responsible for 30 percent of the risk of obesity, while others say 70 percent. But all agree that the real answer is how our genes express themselves, and that is based on what is happening in our environment.

When we starve ourselves on yo-yo diets, eat processed foods, surround ourselves with toxins, work beyond the point of exhaustion, all of these choices influence the way our metabolisms process food, burn calories, and regulate weight. To learn how to use this plan to manipulate our biochemistry to our benefit, we have to understand how our hormones have already been manipulated to our detriment.

One warning: Some of the stuff you'll read here isn't going to be pretty. But we have to know what we're up against before we can fight back.

ENDOCRINE DISRUPTORS: A SEARCH-AND-DESTROY MISSION

You now know that your metabolism is made up of different hormones. When these hormones are functioning normally, everything's just fine—your muscles use appropriate amounts of blood sugar, your insulin stays stable, your thyroid hums along normally. Everything is in balance, burning off energy as you take it in.

But when those hormone levels start getting funky and one goes south, the rest scratch their heads and go, "Huh?" Then they try to sort things out for themselves. Each gland starts over- or underproducing its hormone in a desperate attempt to get back to homeostasis. And that's when the pounds pile on. Any factor that gets in the way of your body's normal hormone functioning spells trouble for your metabolism.

An endocrine disruptor is any substance or influence that somehow alters the way the body's hormones usually work. They may increase, decrease, or change the normal activity of hormones in a number of ways, including

- Mimicking a hormone and clicking into a receptor, setting it off as if it were the hormone itself
- Blocking a real hormone from having access to its receptor
- Increasing or decreasing the number of hormone receptors in certain parts of the body
- Changing the amount of a specific hormone that's produced
- Impacting the speed at which the hormones are processed in the body

Any of these actions can set up a chain of events. For example, let's say your body absorbs bisphenol A, a chemical that's been shown to leach out of polycarbonate plastic containers into the liquids they hold. Studies on animals have found that those exogenous estrogens zoom into the body and, within as little as thirty minutes, decrease blood sugar levels and sharply increase insulin levels. After just four days of exposure, that BPA stimulates the pancreas to secrete more insulin and the body starts to become insulin-resistant.

Now consider the fact that we have more than one thousand additive chemicals in our packaging and food processing. Think of how many other plastics hit your lips or your food in one day—that Styrofoam coffee cup, the squeeze bottle of salad dressing, the cling wrap around your leftovers, the liner in a can of soup, that microwavable bag of vegetables. Think of the scents in your laundry detergent and the chlorine bleach in your bathroom scrub. The ChemLawn truck parked in front of your neighbor's house. The . . .

Can you see how a teeny little problem might start to snowball? This diet and lifestyle program is all about stopping that endocrine-disrupting snowball before it picks up new problems, careens downhill, and destroys everything in its path.

As with nearly everything in our overbloated society, one of the reasons we're getting so fat is because of the way we consume. We purchase in bulk. We want things to be cheap. We want them to last forever on the shelf. All of this comes at a hefty cost to our health. Let's take a look at some of the factors that might set the snowball off on its rapid and destructive descent.

▶ TOO MANY LAZY YEARS

I can't tell you how many people just let exercise slide as they get older, and then turn around and blame their lagging metabolism on their hormones. That's why I want to get the age question out of the way as soon as possible.

A few hormones increase as we get older; others stay the same. But I'll admit it. Most hormones are headed in one direction: south.

Yes, as we age, our hormones shift in ways that encourage weight gain. For example, as you get older, the leptin receptors in your brain start to decrease, so your body doesn't recognize when you're full—which can lead you to overeat. In women, female hormones decrease and insulin-regulating hormones are less effective, both of which can lead to more pounds. For men, bioavailable testosterone levels tend to decline gradually, about 1.5 percent per year after age thirty, and DHEA levels decline even faster—2 to 3 percent per year. These declines can decrease muscle mass and energy while they increase belly fat and insulin resistance. They also make you irritable and depressed—which is all very bad news for your metabolism.

These hormonal declines give drug companies and hormone pushers all the ammunition they need. They use them to support their marketing claims that we need to supplement with synthetic or bioidentical hormones to compensate for the hit to our metabolism or to help extend our lives. But do we really? A major study of more than eleven hundred men aged forty to seventy found that if they maintained a healthy weight, stayed away from excessive drinking, and avoided serious illnesses like diabetes and heart disease, they could add 10 to 15 percent to the levels of several hormones, especially their androgens.

Every day, though, more and more research points to the fact that age-related muscle decline is largely under our control. We've spent years blaming the fat on our bellies on our advancing years, but the truth is, we just haven't been taking care of ourselves! The more we eat clean, live clean, and work out, the better our hormone balance will be, and the healthier our metabolism will remain.

Look, I'll be honest. I don't like to exercise. But the reality is we have to do it. Your body needs it like it needs oxygen and water.

First of all, every pound of muscle burns three times more calories than every pound of fat does. Muscles scoop up blood sugar and enhance your body's insulin sensitivity. Exercise reduces weight-gain hormones like cortisol by releasing endorphins to combat stress and increases fat-burning hormones like testosterone, human growth hormone, DHEA, and thyroxine (T4) production. You need exercise. Period.

(Yes, I know this is not an exercise book, but you can't deny the benefits and the necessities of working out. If you want the information in this diet to be *really* effective, you will work out simultaneously. I am not asking for a grueling fitness regimen. I am simply saying get off your butt and incorporate some healthy activity into your life as soon as possible. I'll talk more about how you can get the most positive impact in the least amount of exercise time in chapter 8.)

Now, if you want to go the route of supplemental hormones, that's a matter for you and your doctor. Do some reading (my favorite book on the subject is *Ageless,* by Suzanne Somers), and talk to a few antiaging endocrinologists. Definitely go to a specialist. Frankly, the research that came out a few years ago in the Women's Health Study about the spike in the risks of heart disease and cancer in women who received hormone replacement therapy scared the crap out of me! But lots of research is ongoing and could uncover some great things in the near future.

In the meantime, I designed this diet to explore other avenues to pro-

tect and optimize hormone balance *naturally* to comply with our bodies'
God-given design. Nature has provided us with the cure; we just keep
messing it up! We have amazing foods—which we'll talk about in chapter 6—that not only help us balance our hormones but also fight cancer,
diabetes, stroke, heart disease, and Alzheimer's. But what do we do? We
spray them with pesticides and toxic gases, turning our natural medicine
into poison. We have to reclaim these natural hormone balancers and
fight back against the many ways our hormones are under assault every
day. I'll show you the simple, safe, natural, and effective strategies that
will help you feel better and help your body cope, without all those nasty
pharmaceuticals.

TOO MANY YO-YO DIETS

If you're reading this book, I'm willing to bet that you've given this weight-
loss thing a go or two in your lifetime. About 75 percent of Americans are
concerned about their weight, but most are not going about addressing it
in the right way. A survey by the International Food Information Council
found that only 15 percent could accurately estimate the number of calories they should be eating for their height and weight.

That lack of knowledge sets us up to fail. People go to crazy extremes
to lose weight. They cut out entire macronutrients, like carbs or fats. This
is all BAD, BAD, BAD. This type of dieting directly disrupts your hormone balance, sending survival messages to the body to store fat and
slow down your metabolism in case the state of famine persists.

Most "weight cyclers"—aka yo-yo dieters—have been on diets all
their life. This pattern of eating starts as early as the teen years. One
study done at the University of Minnesota tracked twenty-five hundred
teens—both boys and girls—for five years and found that those who dieted were three times more likely to be overweight and six times more
likely to be binge eaters than their peers who'd never dieted. The Nurses'
Health Study found that severe weight cyclers, those who'd lost at least
twenty pounds three times within the past four years, gained an average
of ten pounds more than women who'd maintained a more stable weight.
Weight cyclers typically prefer to "diet" to lose weight as opposed to eating proper portions of the right foods. This becomes an even bigger problem when paired with a lack of exercise.

Not only is this up-and-down pattern frustrating, it makes each weight-loss attempt more frustrating than the one before—especially if you lost weight by starving your body. You have to work out when you diet to maintain your muscle mass. This "calorie partitioning" ensures that the calories you do consume go toward rebuilding and repairing your muscles.

If you don't work out, once the diet is over, it becomes apparent pretty quickly that you've just screwed yourself. Starvation diets are catabolic; they prompt your body to cannibalize your muscles for fuel. Your body, wisely, is thinking about long-term survival and wants to hold on to all the calories it can in case of a prolonged famine. Without that muscle, your metabolism is slower, plus your powerful metabolic thyroid hormones are lowered. And the most significant change in thyroid and resting metabolic rate comes when people make the most drastic cuts in their calories.

So many people I've worked with got themselves into a fast/slip-up/ binge pattern. You desperately want to lose pounds for the big day and figure a couple of weeks of eight hundred calories a day can do only good things. What happens? Well, first of all, your metabolism downgrades itself incredibly fast. Then you go back to what would be considered normal eating of roughly sixteen hundred to two thousand calories a day, and you're toast. Your T3 levels have plummeted. Your sensitivity to leptin and insulin has taken a hit. Your ghrelin has shot through the roof. And on and on it goes.

TOO MANY OF THE SAME FOODS, ALL PROCESSED

Some foods, especially processed foods, are murder on our hormone balance. Why? Here's the dirty little secret: Our bodies don't recognize them as foods.

Processed foods don't come from nature; they come from factories. The more productive the factories, the more money the corporation makes. And the less the corporation can spend on the cheap raw materials going into those factories, the higher the profit margins. Well, who can blame them? Higher profits, higher productivity—isn't that the American way? Put pennies in, take dollars out. That must get kind of addictive. Kind of like the "foods" they're creating.

Our twenty-first-century diet is composed primarily of corn, soy, and wheat—whether or not we ever consciously recognize them on our plates. These crops have been subsidized for so long, and have become so inexpensive for food manufacturers, that they're constantly trying to figure out new ways to use these cheap ingredients. And through the miracle of modern chemistry, food manufacturers essentially do just that. You may think you're about to eat a piece of lunch meat/bowl of soup/glass of juice, but it is really basically wheat, soy, or corn. Refined wheat flour. Hydrolyzed soy protein. Partially hydrogenated corn oil. High-fructose corn syrup. With a bit of salt thrown in, too. (Another cheap additive.)

How do they do that? How do they get us to eat these three foods in everything? Well, food manufacturers take these three incredibly cheap, incredibly bland ingredients and add a whole mélange of chemicals to make them actually have taste. Think of corn, soy, and wheat as the blank canvas upon which the food-science industry paints the *illusion* of food. And to keep the illusion going, they may even be resorting to dirty tricks.

Foods high in fat and sugar make the brain release "endogenous opioids," aka biological morphine. If you've ever thought of an Oreo, made up of nearly 60 percent sugar and fat, as a drug you had a jones for, you were right on the money. Just like when an addict is reminded of his drug, your brain's orbitofrontal cortex, the center of motivation and cravings, is stimulated when you see, smell, or taste foods you crave.

Yes, people, we can get high on dessert and we can get addicted. "Well, you could just say no," say the people arguing for "personal responsibility." But here's where the story gets a bit tricky. A 2005 investigative series from the *Chicago Tribune* reported that Kraft, the makers of the Oreo cookie, had shared brain research with scientists from Philip Morris, the tobacco company, and Miller Brewing, the beer maker, all corporate partners at the time. (Hmm, cigarettes, alcohol, and Oreos . . . what could they possibly have in common?) When the *Tribune* broke the story, the Kraft spokesperson said it was just good business to have their scientists "look for ways to exchange information, share *best practices* [italics are mine], and identify efficiencies that reduce overall costs."

Interesting, huh?

Bottom line? The more processed the food is, the greater the chance is

ARE YOU A FOOD ADDICT?

When people see their favorite foods, the neurochemical associated with pleasure, dopamine, is released into the area of the brain linked to motivation and rewards. Just like junkies, obese people have fewer dopamine receptors in this area—and the more obese they are, the fewer receptors they have. Scientists aren't sure if the receptors get worn out from repeated dopamine baths brought on by drug or food binges, or if addicts are born with fewer receptors to begin with, but the net effect is the same—they're constantly left wanting *more*. Strategies that help boost dopamine naturally—like working out or eating enough protein—can help.

that some unscrupulous biochemist is tinkering around with your neuro-chemistry to make you want to eat more—and more and more. We'll talk about how toxic processed foods are to your hormones and overall health in chapter 5, but for now, just realize that as long as the combination of low-quality starch + sugar + fat + salt + addictive chemicals is the cheapest and most profitable combination for megafood corporations, they're going to fight like crazy to keep it on the shelves and in our mouths. Until our government can learn to listen to the research and stand up to the food lobbies, and make this widespread poisoning of the public more expensive for them, we have to figure out how to protect ourselves. And *Master Your Metabolism* will help you do that!

▶ TOO MANY PESTICIDES IN OUR FOOD

Most of the crops food manufacturers are getting their "main" ingredients from are genetically modified or sprinkled with dozens of endocrine-disrupting pesticides. Our buddy corn is one of the worst offenders: The Organic Consumers Organization reported that every year, the corn fed to animals and turned into other corn products is sprayed with 162 million pounds of chemical pesticides. We have no idea what's going into our bodies, and it shows.

A recent large-scale epidemiological study by the National Institutes of Health looked at what happened to thirty thousand people, mostly men, who used pesticides in their work on farms. These "licensed applicators" of the chemicals probably had protective gear—goggles, gloves, boots, overalls—the whole nine yards. Yet researchers found that if these men used any one of seven specific pesticides—even if they used them just once—they had a much greater risk of diabetes. The results suggest that being exposed to pesticides may be a significant contributing factor to diabetes, just like obesity, lack of exercise, or a family history.

One of these pesticides, trichlorfon, is a popular product often used on lawns and golf courses. This study found that people who had used this chemical just ten or more times had a nearly *250 percent greater chance* of developing diabetes. Now, I ask you: How many rounds of golf have you played in your lifetime? How many times has the ChemLawn truck parked in front of your neighbor's house? Or your own?

Now consider our diet. As consumers, we're not only touching plants with pesticides on them—we're *eating* them. In some parts of the world, trichlorfon is even poured over cattle to treat them for pests.

Some pesticides that have been banned in the States for more than twenty years are still hanging around in our food supply. They accumulate in the fatty tissues of our bodies and stick with us for decades. They're found in fish, birds, other mammals, human breast milk. The CDC says we get exposed to organochlorines, a family of toxic chemicals found in pesticides, through

- Eating fatty foods, such as milk, dairy products, or fish, that are contaminated with these pesticides
- Eating foods imported from countries that still allow use of these pesticides
- Breast-feeding or through the placenta when we are in utero
- Our skin

Some researchers argue that pesticides may be more to blame for insulin resistance, metabolic syndrome, and diabetes than obesity is! One study of more than two thousand adults found that at least 80 percent had detectable levels of six "persistent organic pollutants," or POPs, chemicals that remain in our tissues for up to ten years, possibly more. Those people whose bodies had high levels of POPs such as dioxin, PCBs, and chlordane were *thirty-eight times more likely* to be insulin-resistant than people with low levels. Even people who were fatter but didn't have any traces of POPs in their systems had much lower rates of diabetes.

I'm not saying pesticides are the only cause of diabetes. But it's clear that the POPs in your body fat continue to interact with the excess pounds to drive up your diabetes risk even further.

I didn't even mention the organochlorines' other fun side effects—tremors, headaches, skin irritations, breathing problems, dizziness, nausea, seizures. Oh, and cancer, brain damage, Parkinson's disease, birth defects, respiratory illness, abnormal immune system function . . . Shall I go on?

And think of it—organochlorines are just one category of chemical pesticides, just a small sliver of the endocrine-disrupting potential that lurks in the entire food supply. We also have pregnancy and lactation hormones given to dairy cattle to "improve yield." Or growth hormones given to cattle to create more meat. Or antibiotics injected into chickens wedged into shoebox cages to prevent the spreading of illnesses. As terrifying as some of the research is, scientists still mostly just look at each of these chemicals, pesticides, and other endocrine disruptors one at a time, in isolation. New research suggests that the combined, synergistic effect of all of these substances may be way worse than we could possibly imagine.

Whenever I talk about eating organic food, some people always wonder what the fuss is about. "C'mon—is the extra money *really* worth it, Jillian? Times are tough."

What price do you put on your health? Why are women getting breast cancer in their early thirties? Why are we putting eight-year-olds on statins? Why are mysterious diseases like fibromyalgia popping up over the last ten years seemingly out of nowhere? Are you not as scared as I am?

When you ask about the extra money for organics, how much do you think all those prescriptions for obesity-related diseases are going to cost? Or chemotherapy? Lots, I bet. I know people who have lost their homes because of illness. Every dollar you put into prevention will save you thousands down the road in treatment.

Think of this: We get the highest concentration of organic pollutants from our food when we are between one and five years old, just as our obesity genes are being switched on or off, just as our metabolic patterns are being set. We've endured this toxic onslaught for years without knowing what it's doing to our bodies. Now that we know, we *must* start paying very close attention to where our food comes from. I am not being an alarmist when I say that every bite could have lifelong ramifications on our health, hormones, and metabolism.

▶ TOO MANY TOXINS IN OUR ENVIRONMENT

Our food is not the only place riddled with endocrine-disrupting toxins. More than one hundred thousand synthetic chemicals have been registered for commercial use—with two thousand more added each year—but very few of them have been tested adequately for toxicity, let alone for any potential hormonal activity. Instead, officials have pooh-poohed their effects. "These things are dangerous only at very high levels," they say, neglecting to mention that they didn't test them at very low levels. Now researchers are starting to realize that many of these chemicals impact our endocrine systems at moderate and even *minute* levels. And they're starting to pile up in our bodies. Research on Swedish women found that the concentration of polybrominated diphenyl ether (aka the flame retardants found in baby pajamas, pillow cases, electronics, and furniture) in their breast milk doubled every five years from 1972 to 1998.

And this stuff really messes with our hormones. Take the women who fish in Lake Ontario, which is known to have high levels of polychlorinated biphenyls (PCBs). A study in the *American Journal of Epidemiology* found that the fisherwomen who ate more than one fish meal a month for several years had shorter menstrual cycles than women who didn't. Other studies on women who eat fish from PCB-laden lakes suggest they have a harder time getting pregnant.

Girlie bits aren't the only ones affected. Boy rats exposed to just one dose of dioxin in the womb produced 74 percent fewer sperm than those that had not been exposed. Their levels of testosterone were lower than normal, and the size of their genitals was significantly reduced. The researchers said it was clear that prenatal exposure to dioxin "demasculinizes and feminizes male rats." (I don't know too many guys who want their junk shrunk, do you?)

Some studies have also shown that when animals are subjected to PCBs and dioxins, their thyroid glands change in ways similar to the way people react to Hashimoto's disease. When pregnant rats are exposed to increased levels of PCBs, their babies have less thyroid hormone and wacky neurotransmitter levels. Carbon tetrachloride, a chemical sometimes found in drinking-water tests, has been linked to thyroid dysfunction. Researchers are also beginning to see that fish in lakes and rivers are actually getting chemically induced sex changes—boys are becoming girls—because of the high levels of man-made estrogens in the water!

These xenoestrogens are endangering us at all levels of life. In April 2008, Canada became the first country to ban bisphenol A, or BPA, a chemical that's been shown to mimic estrogen in the body, from baby bottles. After Canadian officials reviewed the available research, they decided that the risks were too great to allow babies to ingest it. Thereafter, an article in the *Journal of the American Medical Association* found that higher BPA concentrations in people's urine were associated with a 300 percent greater risk of cardiovascular disease and a 240 percent greater risk of diabetes, as well as abnormalities in liver enzymes. Women with PCOS have higher blood levels of BPA compared with women who don't have the disease. Even low doses of BPA have been shown to create new fat cells and increase their size. In all, more than 130 animal studies have linked very low doses of BPA to breast and

ENDOCRINE DISRUPTORS ABOUND

This extremely abbreviated list of endocrine-disrupting chemicals in our environment is just the

Chemical	Other Names	Uses
Polychlorinated biphenyls	PCBs	Have been banned since 1977 but were originally used for coolants, electrical equipment, metal cutting oils, microscope lens oils, and in inks, dyes, and carbonless copy paper; might still be found in old fluorescent light fixtures
Phthalates	DEHP, DINP	Added to plastics to make them flexible
Dioxins		Byproduct of incineration and industrial processes
Bisphenol A	BPA	Added to plastics to make them more durable
Volatile organic compounds	VOCs	N/A (VOCs are byproducts with no practical use)
Chlorine	Bleach	Disinfectant; industrial manufacturing ingredient
Nonylphenol ethoxylates	NPEs	"Surfactants," chemical dirt-lifting agents

tip of the iceberg.

You Can Find Them In	Potential or Proven Health Effects
Farm raised salmon, freshwater fish (despite being outlawed for over 30 years)	Severe form of acne (chloracne), swelling of the upper eyelids, discoloring of the nails and skin, numbness in the arms and/or legs, weakness, muscle spasms, chronic bronchitis, problems related to the nervous system, increased incidence of cancer, particularly liver and kidney cancer
Medical tubing, teething rings, pacifiers, shower curtains, plastic wrap, plastic food containers; also used to lengthen the life of fragrances	Reduced sperm counts and decreased fertility in animals
Eating nonorganic animal products (dioxin builds up in fatty tissues)	Lower rate of male births in humans; reduction in sperm counts, production of testosterone, and male genital size in rats; reproductive cancer; developmental disorders; skin rashes, liver damage, excess body hair
Baby bottles, polycarbonate drinking bottles (old Nalgene), interior liners of food and beverage cans	Increased risk of breast and prostate cancer, infertility, PCOS, insulin resistance, and diabetes
Off-gassing from paints, vinyls, plastics, cleaning products, solvents, air fresheners, fabric softener, dryer sheets, wall-to-wall carpeting, deodorant, dry-cleaned clothing, cosmetics	Nausea, headache, drowsiness, sore throat, dizziness, and memory impairment. Long-term exposure can cause cancer. Many products with VOCs also contain phthalates.
Drinking water, industrial waste, household cleaners, chlorine pools, bleached paper (paper towels, coffee filters), nylon	Respiratory problems (wheezing, coughing, constricted airways), lung pain or collapse, eye and skin irritation, sore throat. Heated chlorine creates dioxin.
Household and laundry detergents and other cleaning agents	The Sierra Club reported that these potent gender benders "cause organisms to develop both male and female sex organs; increase mortality and damage to the liver and kidneys; decrease testicular growth and sperm counts in male fish; and disrupt normal male-to-female sex-ratios, metabolism, development, growth, and reproduction." These effects also intensify as NPEs break down in the environment.

prostate cancer, early puberty, brain damage, obesity, diabetes, lowered sperm count, hyperactivity, damaged immune system, and other serious conditions.

The problem is, BPA is everywhere—more than 6 billion pounds of BPA are produced in the world every year, one-third of it by the United States. A CDC study found that 95 percent of Americans have BPA in their urine. Manufacturers add BPA to polycarbonate plastic and the linings of cans, bottles, and other food containers.

These toxic endocrine disruptors in our environment do more than just mess with our metabolisms—they may give us hormonally-influenced cancer. A recent Harvard study found that as many as 50 percent of all prostate cancers are linked to excess estrogen in the body. According to Physicians for Social Responsibility, some of the most common pollutants found in plastics, fuels, drugs, and pesticides cause cancer in animals (and likely in humans) precisely by interfering with healthy hormone activity.

Those of us Gen X- and Yers, who are younger than baby boomers, may be doubly screwed—we didn't have a childhood foundation free of these endocrine disruptors that could've shielded us or at least given us a bit of resistance against some of this. Instead, we've been raised in an environment that essentially has been upping the hormones on all sides, all with the net outcome of making us fat—and unhealthy!

And it's the combination of all of these factors that scares the crap out of me. One report looked at the impact of PCBs and dioxin, both of which were widely detected in people's bodies. The combination of these two chemicals inflicted *four hundred times* as much damage to the liver as dioxin alone. Now multiply that by the number of chemicals out in the environment today.

We have to start protecting ourselves right now!

TOO MANY BAD BUGS—AND NOT ENOUGH GOOD ONES

Part of what lured us into this pesticide-riddled mess was the desire to kill the "pests" that live all around us but seemed bothersome or threatening. We, the superior beings, are certainly entitled to do that, right? We tried to rid ourselves of every bug, big and small, especially scary ones like staph, salmonella, and *E. coli*, with an onslaught of antibacterial products. We pump our livestock full of antibiotics. Heck, we pump ourselves full of antibiotics.

Here's the deal: Trying to get rid of most bacteria is not only dangerous, it's practically pointless. According to an article in the *New York Times,* of the trillions of cells in your body, *only one out of every ten is human.* The rest are bacteria, fungi, protozoa—in total, more than five hundred other species of microbes, most of which are hanging out in your gut.

Most of these bugs are actually beneficial—these "probiotics" that live in our bellies are integral to the healthy functioning of our immune and digestive systems. But when they get out of balance, and the "bad" bugs overwhelm the beneficial bugs, bad things start to happen. You might get yeast infections, diarrhea, or other stomach-bug symptoms. You might develop food allergies. You might succumb to truly evil bugs, such as methicillin-resistant *Staphylococcus aureus,* or MRSA, a potentially fatal staph infection you can pick up in hospitals and other public settings.

You might even get fat.

Dr. Nikhil Dhurandhar created the term "infectobesity" to describe the phenomenon of infection as a cause of obesity. In the past twenty years, at least ten pathogens have been reported to increase weight in humans and animals, including viruses, bacteria, and microflora in the gut.

Researchers at Washington University have found that when people lose weight, the proportion of two key microflora—Bacteriodetes and Firmicutes, which comprise 90 percent of the gut flora—change. These researchers believe that our "gut microbial ecology" may actually be responsible for how many calories our bodies absorb from food and send to fat cells. They first did a study on mice and found that obese mice had 50 percent fewer Bacteriodetes and 50 percent more Firmicutes. Then they did a study on human beings and found that as people lost weight, either on a low-fat or low-carb diet, their skinny Bacteriodetes started flourishing and the fat Firmicutes diminished. The researchers believe Firmicutes bacteria actually help the body absorb more calories, especially from carbs, and send more directly into fat. But as the people lost weight, it's almost as if they shed these bacteria in favor of the leaner, meaner Bacteriodetes. The researchers even wondered if perhaps some people are predisposed to obesity because they start out with a higher proportion of Firmicutes in their intestines.

The irony is that when you take antibiotics to help wipe out the "bad" bacteria, you end up taking out the "good" bacteria, your best defense, at the same time. Then you have to start building up your beneficial bacteria's defenses again, a nearly impossible challenge when fed solely on the standard diet of processed foods that the "bad" bacteria adore. The only thing we can do is to keep our immune systems strong and take care of our microflora environments by eating the kinds of foods that replenish and feed our beneficial bacteria so they can counterbalance the activity of the negative bacteria. This plan helps you by focusing on organic meat and dairy from animals that have been raised without the use of antibiotics, and by avoiding overmedicating your body with antibiotics whenever possible.

▶ TOO MANY HOURS AT WORK—AND NOT ENOUGH IN BED

Stress is like kryptonite for your hormones—even just a bit of it can throw them entirely out of whack. If you remain a stress case for a long time, you could do some major damage to many parts of your body, including your glands. (Just think of how I screwed up my thyroid with years of cortisol overload, calorie deprivation, and overall general abuse.)

According to Dr. Scott Isaacs, author of *The Leptin Boost Diet* and guru of all things hormonal, stress can cause

- Leptin resistance
- Insulin resistance
- Lower estrogen (estradiol) in women
- Lower testosterone in men
- Lower levels of growth hormone
- Higher cortisol levels
- Impaired conversion of thyroid hormone

Every single one of these hormonal changes will slow down your metabolism and cause you to gain weight. Add them together, and then throw in all the behavioral issues that come with stress—eating on the run, stress snacking, eating at night, not exercising, excess caffeine and/or alcohol, even a stolen cigarette or two—and you will see that stress is a major source of endocrine disruption.

Perhaps one of the biggest causes and symptoms of the hormonal shutdown from stress is when people start to cut into their hours of quality sleep. The percentage of young adults sleeping eight to nine hours per night has almost been cut in half in the past fifty years, from 40 percent in 1960 to 23 percent in 2002. During the same time period, the incidence of obesity has nearly doubled. Coincidence?

A study done at the University of Chicago found that when a group of young men had their sleep restricted just two nights in a row, their levels of the satiety hormone leptin dropped almost 20 percent, and their levels of the hunger hormone ghrelin shot up almost 30 percent—in short, they became ravenous. Their appetite for sweet foods (like candy, cookies, and ice cream) and starchy foods (like bread and pasta) shot up 33 percent, and for salty foods (like chips and salted nuts), 45 percent. Left to their own devices, these guys would've wolfed down almost twice as many carbohydrates as before the study. Other research from the same institution found that when healthy people were deprived of the ability to reach deep, slow-wave sleep—the period in which most of our growth hormone is released—for just three days, their ability to process sugar dropped by 23 percent. They essentially became insulin-resistant in just seventy-two hours.

We need our rest!

TOO MANY PHARMACEUTICALS—EVEN IN OUR WATER

Drugs are big business. And drug companies have become very creative about selling us sickness via new lifestyle diseases. Whether you're sad, anxious, mad, hyper, or feel any other human emotion, they have a drug to medicate it away. Here's my favorite: restless leg syndrome. I mean, really?! And despite the fact that women have been going through menopause for thousands upon thousands of years, now we need drugs to manage that as well?

Here's one that I played around with and paid the price for: Accutane. When I was in my twenties, I had acne. So I did what any vain twenty-something would do—I went to a dermatologist and asked for Accutane. I didn't know what it would do to me; I just didn't want to break out anymore. Nobody explained to me how serious its side effects could be. I'm convinced—though my dermatologist argues with me about it to this day—that I became more estrogen-dominant because taking it helped shut down my testosterone production. And my endocrinologist agrees with me! To add insult to injury, after I took the Accutane, I started to develop the melasma on my face. While it may have been due in part to increased sensitivity to sunlight, abnormal facial pigmentation is also an unmistakable sign of estrogen dominance.

Now, you expect your hormones are going to get tossed around a bit when you're on birth control pills or hormone replacement therapy. But skin medication? And that's just the start of it. Even if you leave aside the obvious hormonal actions, many pharmaceuticals have been found to have endocrine-disrupting chemicals in them as well. A common class of antidepressants, selective serotonin reuptake inhibitors, or SSRIs, has been linked to higher rates of metabolic syndrome. And a French study found that after only four to six weeks on the antipsychotic medicine olanzapine, animals had higher blood sugar levels and more fat around their bellies.

One major review found that many classes of pharmaceuticals cause weight gain:

Anticonvulsants
Antidiabetics
Antihistamines
Antihypertensives
Contraceptives
HIV antiretroviral drugs and protease inhibitors
Psychotropics (antipsychotics, antidepressants, mood stabilizers)
Steroid hormones (such as prednisone)

All of these pharmaceuticals could have a serious impact on your hormonal health. Because our medical system doesn't think holistically, your doctor could prescribe one drug to help you achieve the desired results in one part of your system, while over in another, you're throwing a hormone level totally out of whack. Certain herbs, vitamins, and other supplements can have very powerful hormonal effects. If your doctor doesn't know you're taking them, and dashes off another prescription in haste, you could do real damage to your endocrine system.

You say you never take pharmaceuticals or any other pills, so this particular endocrine disruptor won't apply to you? Think again. The Associated Press did a massive study on the municipal water supplies of fifty of the country's major metropolitan areas. They found that twenty-four of them—

the water supply of 41 million Americans—had detectable levels of pharmaceuticals. At least one, Philadelphia's, had *fifty-six different drugs,* including antibiotics, anticonvulsants, mood stabilizers, and sex hormones.

How did all those pharmaceuticals get there? Several ways, but mainly through our toilets. How gross is that?

This drug-addled drinking water not only comes from human waste. Livestock that are fed or injected with hormones or antibiotics will also pee or poop them out, and they'll leach into the groundwater. Some of the hormones given to cattle can be one hundred to one thousand times stronger in biological activity than other environmental hormone disruptors.

The wastewater is treated at several stages, but many drugs remain because no sewage treatments were designed to remove them. Only reverse osmosis removes almost all pharmaceutical residue, but don't hold your breath that your local water authority will start using that process—it's too expensive for large-scale use. (Which is why in chapter 8 I recommend that you install a reverse osmosis filter in your home.)

No one knows exactly what decades of drinking this medicated water will do to us, but disturbing trends are popping up all over nature. One study found that fish swimming in rivers downstream from a cattle farm had four times the hormonal activity of those swimming upstream.

▶ TOO MANY CIGARETTES

A *Journal of Endocrinology* review of more than one hundred studies on the hormonal effect of smoking came to a stunning conclusion: Smoking sucks.

Smoking impacts many endocrine glands—your pituitary, thyroid, adrenals, testicles, ovaries—in addition to your lungs, heart, brain, and, oh yeah, every other cell in your body. Smoking helps cause insulin resistance and diabetes, drives up your cortisol levels, and gives you a fat stomach. Smoking can make you infertile and throw your body into menopause years before your time. Smoking is also a huge risk factor in developing problems with your thyroid—it can lead to hypothyroidism because of increases in levels of thiocyanate, a known goitrogen (a substance that grows goiters). If you're already hypothyroid, smoking cuts your thyroid secretion even further.

Even with all we know about smoking, I still have twenty-year-olds who come to me, smoking like chimneys, saying, "I can't quit—I don't want to get fat!" (In fact, a survey of four thousand women in *Self* magazine found that 13 percent of women smoke to lose weight.)

I have news for you—smoking will *make you* fat. And old. And ugly. Oh, and maybe dead. That's hardly a sustainable beauty regimen.

Do we really have to go over this? For the last time, people, quit smoking. Just because some starlet is shown chain-smoking her heart out at a sidewalk café doesn't mean that's the secret behind her weight-loss plan. Smoking fills your body with many pollutants that not only won't help you lose weight, they will make you fat.

Just don't do it.

TOO MUCH, PERIOD!

This last reason our hormones are in full meltdown mode is often one of the first reasons cited for our excess pounds: the "obesogenic environment." And yes, there's no denying that we are struggling with an environment that conspires to make and keep us fat. Restaurant portions have increased up to 500 percent since the 1970s. On average, we each eat 23 pounds of candy and drink 35 gallons of regular soda a year. Add in remote controls, no sidewalks, 5 million television channels, Internet addictions, drive-throughs, longer commutes, extended workweeks, super sizing. . . . Okay, I can see you starting to nod off.

You've heard this.

You know this.

You've read all about "portion creep" and all the other insidious ways our food supply has ballooned over the years.

But we have to see this epidemic of "too much" not just as a harmless symptom of our supposedly greedy appetites. I want you to see this caloric excess as a highly profitable, corporately sanctioned endocrine disruptor every bit as scary and horrific as the pesticides and pharmaceuticals we talked about earlier. I want you to look at supersized, overblown fast foods and think of them as bordering on grotesque, just like the thought of swallowing a glass full of estrogen right out of your tap. We need to look at these huge portions as poisonous in and of themselves, to help us realize that by cutting back, we're not depriving ourselves—we're sidestepping an enormous black hole of toxins in our environment.

And we *can* fight back; there are hopeful signs everywhere of how we can change our country's zombie walk straight into the deep-fat fryer. One study found that if schools offered kids in fourth to sixth grade healthier snacks (and rewards for eating them), limited the availability of soda and junk foods, and provided fifty hours of nutrition education per year (woven into the normal curriculum), they reduced the number of overweight kids by 50 percent, compared with a control school that took none of these steps.

If they can do it in school, you can do it in your house. Toss the soda, keep reading about nutrition—i.e., this book!—and follow this plan back to a place where your metabolism and hormones start working for you, instead of greedy corporate poison peddlers.

OKAY, GUYS, DON'T PANIC

When you look at all of these factors together, it's kind of unbelievable that everyone isn't morbidly obese. We are locked in a struggle, there's no doubt about it. But once we've had our eyes opened, we can start to do things differently. Each change you make here will make a positive difference in your endocrine function and create changes of its own. Soon you'll have a much healthier, more balanced endocrine system—and a lot less fat to show for it. Now let's take a look at how we'll accomplish just that.

CHAPTER 4

HOW THE DIET WORKS

OVERVIEW OF HOW THE REMOVE/RESTORE/REBALANCE
PLAN RESETS YOUR METABOLISM

Now that you know what you're up against, you may feel like throwing up your hands and saying, "Forget it. The deck is stacked against me. I can't possibly fight back!"

But you can.

What you need is a plan. A program. A systematic way of fending off the assaults on your endocrine system, no matter where they may be coming from. A science-based approach that will recalibrate your hormonal levels, so you can be healthy and reset your metabolism to do what it was meant to do: burn calories and shed fat.

So how are we going to do that? Simple, really. We're going to come at this in three steps. You're going to Remove the toxins from your diet and your environment; Restore the nutrients to your food and supplement plan; and Rebalance the energy that goes into and comes out of your body. Just these three steps will be all most people need to trigger the fat-burning hormones, quiet down those fat-storing hormones, and get your body back to being a lean, mean machine.

STEP 1: REMOVE

In chapter 3, you heard about the absolutely horrific amount of toxicity in our food and environment. We've talked about how some of these toxins have disrupted our endocrine systems, damaged our metabolisms, made us sick, made us look older and feel less vital, and also, yes, made us fat. We have to get as far away from this crap as we possibly can! When you think of the ten thousand chemicals that we already have on the shelf, and the two thousand more added each year, we need to eliminate as much as possible from our diets and our lives, and keep holding the line.

Step 1 will walk you through your entire kitchen and pantry and help you get rid of the biggest endocrine offenders. Certain endocrine evils you may have already heard of: High-fructose corn syrup? Gone. Hydrogenated oils? Gone. But we'll also talk about some other healthy-sounding foods you may not realize are routinely messing with your hormones. (Who ever thought "spices" could be a bad thing?)

Once we've trashed all the CRAP from your diet, all the foods that encourage your hormones to store fat, we can start to rebuild it with foods that will trigger your fat-*burning* hormones. And that's where Step 2 comes in, Restore.

STEP 2: RESTORE

Before you start thinking that this diet is all about what you can't eat, let's get right to the good stuff. I want you to eat how nature intended us to eat. More important is that I want you to eat foods that will flick the on switch to your metabolism. You will eat foods that will repair, nourish, and support every cell in your body so your body will work for you and not against you. Be good to your body and it will be good to you. And I promise you, after two weeks on this diet, you will never want to go back to that processed, chemical-laden crap again.

In the immortal words of Michael Pollan, author of *The Omnivore's Dilemma,* I want you to "Eat food." That's it! Simple, real, naturally occurring food. Food that has been on this planet for tens of thousands of years. In other words, not foods that say, "Exciting new flavors!" on their labels. Aside from those teeny, annoying labels that always get stuck to fruits and vegetables, you won't be seeing too many labels on this diet.

If I had to sum up Step 2 in one sentence, it would be: "If it didn't have a mother and it didn't grow from the ground, don't eat it." Cheetos don't have a mother and, I don't know about you, I don't recall seeing a Cheeto tree in my backyard when I was growing up.

How do we do this? The biggest part of Step 2 is actually quite simple, and you've likely heard a lot about it. GO ORGANIC. While even organic food is not 100 percent "pure," it is by far the best defense we have against endocrine disruptors in our food supply.

Now, I know some of you are probably bellyaching right now. "Sure, Jillian—easy for you to say! You have the money to do it; I only wish I could afford to eat organic." Here's the deal—you do have the money. If you have a hundred dollars a week for groceries, you have the money. Stop wasting money on gossip rags and junk you don't need and invest that extra cash in your health. We're not going for perfection, we're going for maximum impact. That's why I'll share tons of tools for how to eat organic on a budget, let you know what the biggest chemical culprits in our food supply are, and show you how following a few other Remove rules will actually save you a lot of cash—dollars you can put directly into your organic-produce budget.

You'll eat simple, real, naturally occurring food. Organically grown fruits and vegetables. Grass-fed beef. Organic free-range chicken. Ocean-caught fish. Whole grains. Nuts, beans, seeds. These are foods your body recognizes from way back. In fact, your body knows what to do with every part of these foods, what nutrients get sent to what part of the body, and, most important, what foods turn on (or off) which hormones. These foods make sense to your body.

Imagine spending your whole life speaking one language—you can read, tell jokes, sing songs. You're fluent. Then one day, you wake up and everyone is speaking another language, and they don't understand a word you're saying. You simply can't communicate.

Eating faux foods is like force-feeding your body gibberish and expecting it to understand you. Your body wants to understand the foods you feed it, really and truly. But it can't. So it will be forced to make do, create work-arounds, flub a couple of sentences, use wild hand signals. And try as your body might, it will never be fluent in faux food language, so all those work-arounds will eventually start to pile up and create one giant mess of your biochemisty. And what you're left with is a failure to communicate. And that failure manifests itself in premature aging, disease, obesity, depression, and more.

In Restore, we'll simplify the conversation. We'll get fluent in body language and really listen to the cues we're getting. Your body will say, "Oh, I get it! Now I'm supposed to stop eating!" or "That's right—now I'm supposed to burn these calories, not store them." When you Restore real foods to your diet, you'll talk directly to your genes and your hormones and guide them to do what they're meant to do—maintain your weight and overall health, and add years of quality to your life.

► STEP 3: REBALANCE

Like I said, I want you to eat. Seriously. Three square meals and one snack. That's the only way you're going to convince your hormones that they don't have to hang on to that fat for a rainy day.

Once you're eating the foods that your body recognizes, and there are no funky endocrine disruptors trying to confuse your hormones and trick them into hoarding fat, your body needs to know that there is plenty where that came from. No shortage here. No way you're ever, ever going to run out of food.

Now, before you belly up to the buffet, remember one thing. I've said it a million times, I'll say it again: Calories. Do. Count.

That said, did you ever stop to think about how few calories there are in real food? Apple: 76 calories. Chicken breast: 142 calories. Head of broccoli—yes, the whole head: 135 calories.

Now let's contrast that three-ounce portion of chicken with, oh, say, three ounces of Cheetos: 480 calories. This snack "food" is full of 30 grams of fat, 45 grams of carbs, and more than a third of your daily sodium—as well as half a dozen known endocrine disruptors.

Is it any wonder that kind of "food" is unrecognizable to the human body? There is literally nothing in there that our bodies recognize. So, with faux foods, not only are you putting hundreds of extra calories into your body, you're also feeding your hormones all kinds of mixed signals that will multiply this caloric effect exponentially.

When you Rebalance, you'll see that eating every four hours during the day is best for your body. We'll even talk about how to time your first and last meals of the day to get the very best fat-burning power out of your early-morning and late-night hormonal swings. And you'll learn that eating before you are hungry will make your metabolism start to hum along like a finely tooled machine. Listening to your body and stopping before you're overfull will get easier and easier with practice—and, in time, you'll find out that being "stuffed" isn't comfortable or enjoyable. That Real Food does not exclude any nutrient—carbs, fat, or protein—because hormonal balance (not to mention efficient, safe, permanent weight loss) is possible only when *all* nutrients are present and accounted for.

Now, that covers the "energy in" portion of the Rebalance step—but what about the "energy out"? You know how much I push exercise. I'm a pusher, it's true—guilty as charged. But the "energy out" I'm talking about here is a different kind of energy. I could call it "metaphysical energy" but I don't want to seem too New Age-y. So let's call it the energy you have to do the things you want to do in life. How are you using that energy? How are you protecting that energy? How is that energy impacting your family and friends, job, or love life? How are you recharging and rebalancing that energy? You might be surprised to learn how much the use of your personal energy impacts your hormone levels and your metabolism. How much you sleep, how much you stress and freak out and pull your hair out, how much you, yes, sit on your butt—all of those choices about how you Rebalance your energy stores will directly impact how you rebalance your hormone levels, your weight, and your entire life.

I know you want to Rebalance. We all do. And with the information in this book, you can.

PART 2

THE MASTER PLAN

CHAPTER 5

STEP 1—REMOVE

ELIMINATE THE ANTINUTRIENTS THAT TRIGGER YOUR FAT-STORING HORMONES

Your poor body is stumbling around, trying to scrounge something nutritious out of this toxic food environment. Your willpower is not enough to sustain your weight-loss efforts, because there's too much static. Too many additives and processes have mangled the food supply and confused your body's normal metabolism.

That's why, again, I could sum up this entire food plan in one sentence: *If it didn't have a mother or it didn't grow from the ground, don't eat it.*

I'm sure PETA's going to be after me about that one. But I'm not joking. I'm talking about whole foods. Food the way nature intended, before it got sent to a chem lab and became indecipherable to our biology.

My standard diet used to look something like this:

Breakfast: low-carb protein bar, coffee with NutraSweet
Snack: Diet Coke
Lunch: Diet Coke, 2 slices of low-carb white "bread" with 3 slices of processed turkey
Snack: Diet Coke, processed nonfat cheese with diet crackers
Dinner: nonorganic chicken loaded with antibiotics and nonorganic veggies

Now, looking at that mouth-watering menu, do you think my body was saying, "Ooooh, great, I just ingested tons of trans fats, sugar alcohols, high-fructose corn syrup, nitrates, antibiotics, pesticides, and artificial sweeteners. I know just what to do with this. I'll build some healthy muscle and some smooth skin with it!'"?

No. When I ate this supposedly edible wealth of chemicals, my body got confused. That "food" was basically foreign matter. Check out this ingredient list from the protein bar alone:

Protein blend (soy protein nuggets, [soy protein isolate, rice starch, brown rice flour], whey protein isolate, calcium caseinate), yogurt coating (maltitol/lactitol, palm kernel oil, calcium caseinate, nonfat yogurt powder, palm oil, soy lecithin, titanium dioxide color, oligofructose, fructose, acesulfame K), maltitol, lemon pieces (inulin, fractionated palm kernel oil, oat fiber, citrus oil, citric acid, soy lecithin, acesulfame K, turmeric extract (color), glycerin, cocoa butter, natural and artificial flavor, vitamin and mineral blend (dicalcium phosphate, magnesium oxide, ascorbic acid, d-Alpha tocopheryl acetate, niacinamide, zinc oxide, dextrose, copper gluconate, d-Calcium pantothenate, Vitamin A palmitate, pyridoxine hydrochloride, thiamin mononitrate, riboflavin, folic acid, biotin, potassium iodide, sodium selenite, cyanocobalamin), high oleic sunflower oil, gum, corn syrup solids, citric acid, soy lecithin, potassium sorbate, sucralose. May contain traces of peanuts and/or tree nuts.

Impressive, no? Quite a feat of modern chemical engineering.

(It's funny that the allergen alert about peanuts and tree nuts includes two of the only whole foods on the list.)

News flash: Your body does not jump for joy over this little bomb of toxic chemicals. It scratches its head and goes, "Huh? What the . . . ? Okay, I guess I'll just do . . . *this*."

And "this," your body's very next reaction, is *always, always* bad news to your hormones.

This protein bar is one example. But the same number of processed and chemical ingredients—and sometimes many more—are in other "healthy" cereals, breads, soups, waffles, soy-based meat replacements, and so on. How many times have your eyes glazed over as you tried to decipher an ingredients list with dozens of syllables?

A few manufacturers are consciously trying to break this cycle by using fewer and more natural ingredients. (For a list of some of my favorite brands, check out the Resources on page 243.) But overall, to escape the chemical infestation and hormonal devastation of our food supply, we need to just say, "NO!"

That's why the first part of this diet has to be about what we Remove. If we don't get some of this crap out of your mouth and out of your system, no amount of whole, healthy food will make a dent.

What are we removing? Processed foods get the big no. No chemicals, no MSG. No trans fats. No artificial sweeteners. No additives that "thicken," or "stabilize," or otherwise tamper with the texture or freshness of the food. You're going to learn how to dump the foods that prevent the release of weight-loss hormones. You're also going to learn which foods provoke a rapid release of weight-gain hormones. We'll also remove, or at least reduce, a few whole foods that tend to screw with our hormones, even though they grow from the ground.

Let's take a look at some of the common antinutrients in the modern food supply that most violently disrupt your body's natural biochemistry. The corporations have made some of these antinutrients downright addictive—that's why I want to give you as much motivation to resist them as possible.

▶ PROCESSED FOODS: THE BIG NO

We are a busy nation. We don't have time to cook, let alone get to the market every day—we have stuff to do! So we think, "We need to stock up, buy in bulk, shop once a week."

That's how processed food came to take over the food chain: Corporations figured out a highly profitable way to play off our time deficit. And boy, are we paying for it.

A processed food is any food that's been canned, frozen, dehydrated, or had chemicals added in to make it last longer, texturize it, soften it, allow it to sit on the shelf forever. Some processed foods—like frozen or prechopped veggies—can be a godsend. Maybe not as ideal as buying food in season from a local farmers market, but I'm a realist and whole processed foods help us walk the right path.

What I'm talking about are the processed foods made of refined grains, vegetable oils, and added sugar that comprise almost 60 percent of our diet. We'll get rid of these products that add cheap chemicals and dilute less profitable whole food ingredients—in other words, most of the processed foods we eat!

As you read this section, I want you to grab a trash bag, go through your kitchen and refrigerator, and put this stuff directly into the trash. Sometimes you'll read a diet article that says, "Clean out all your ___ foods and donate them to a soup kitchen or homeless shelter." Forget that! *No one* should eat this food. Why should a poor person eat this crappy food if you shouldn't?

I want you to make the mental connection that this stuff is poison, horrible for your own or anyone else's body. Yes, you may have paid money for it, but cut your losses and also prevent anyone else from poisoning their body. THROW IT AWAY.

ANTINUTRIENT #1: HYDROGENATED FATS

If there are any evil foods in the world, they include hydrogenated fats. Created for the convenience of the processed-foods industry, hydrogenated fats allow foods like chips, crackers, cookies, pies, and bread to sit on the shelf forever and still retain their "freshness." I don't know, is there something wrong with a cookie that can be eaten years after it is produced? *Common sense would probably answer YES to that question.*

Hydrogenated fats are created when a regular fat—such as a corn oil or a palm oil—is blasted with hydrogen to change the liquid into a solid at room temperature. More than any other kind of fat, including saturated fat, hydrogenated fats increase your "bad" LDL and triglycerides and decrease your "good" HDL. They also shrink the size of your LDL particles, which makes them more likely to clot and dramatically raises your risk of heart attack. *Just a 2 percent increase in trans-fatty acids in your diet increases your chance of heart disease by 23 percent.* Eating excess fried foods, which also include trans fats, can increase your risk of metabolic syndrome by 25 percent.

Trans fats also increase your body's inflammation. People who eat more trans fats have higher blood levels of interleukin-6, a hormonelike substance that's been linked to hardening of the arteries, osteoporosis, type 2 diabetes, and Alzheimer's. Research on animals found that interleukin-6-induced inflammation also causes the liver to stop responding to growth hormone and the muscles to wither away—and with that, metabolism. Definitely not the effect we're looking for.

If you make a steady diet of trans fats, heart disease is virtually guaranteed. A *New England Journal of Medicine* review of more than eighty studies found that trans fat is more dangerous to health than any food contaminant, even when it's only 1 to 3 percent of your total calorie intake. The study authors found that you'd need to eat only **20 to 60 calories from artificial trans fats a day to start damaging your health.** And you know how all those chip and cracker companies are claiming "no trans fats" on their packaging? Manufacturers are permitted to use that claim as long as one portion contains less than 500 milligrams of trans fats. A couple of extra smears of your "zero trans fats" margarine and a couple of extra "trans free" cookies can get you over that twenty-calorie mark pretty damn fast.

Hormone Homework: *There is no safe limit to this stuff! Toss out anything with "shortening" or "partially hydrogenated oil" of any type—palm, corn, soybean—as they always include trans fats.*

A small amount of trans fats are also found in meat, created in the bellies of cows, sheep, and goats, but don't worry about these trans fats—they're mainly good guys. These "ruminant" trans fats are not nearly as dangerous as industrially produced trans fats, and may have some health benefits. Research suggests that one, conjugated linoleic acid (CLA), may reduce the risk of breast, prostate, intestinal, lung, and skin cancer, as well as reduce body fat and enhance muscle growth. (Important note: These benefits of CLAs have *not* been demonstrated in supplemental form. In fact, several studies have linked CLA supplements to increased risk of insulin resistance, so please don't supplement with CLAs.)

Hormone Homework: *Always choose organic meats and dairy and look for grass-fed options—cows that are allowed to graze exclusively on grass produce milk and meat with 500 percent more CLAs than those fed grain. (We'll talk a lot about this and many other reasons to choose organics in chapter 6.)*

> ## ANTINUTRIENT #2: REFINED GRAINS

Remember my dictum to eat only food that had a mother or grew from the ground? Once grains are refined, they no longer qualify. Refining grains helps extend their shelf life by removing the bran and the germ of the grain—and with it, almost all the fiber, vitamins, and minerals of the entire grain kernel. And then the B vitamins—thiamin, riboflavin, niacin, folic acid—and the iron stripped out during processing have to be restored by being "enriched." The only people who profit from this process are the corporations who can then stretch these

Want to get rid of fat on your body? Put some more in your mouth. It's true: The party line about reducing dietary fat to decrease body fat is finally losing ground. And not a second too soon— low-fat, high-carbohydrate diets got us into a hormonal mess.

Type	Action/Benefits	Good or Bad
Monounsaturated fatty acids	These fats raise your HDL (high-density lipoprotein), the "good" cholesterol. As your HDL level climbs, your risk of heart disease lowers. Unsaturated fats also lower your levels of LDL (low-density lipoprotein), the "bad" cholesterol that raises your heart disease risk.	Mainly good
Polyunsaturated fatty acids: omega-6s	These fats lower both your HDL and your LDL. Though these were traditionally assumed to be heart-healthy, many sources of these fats (such as corn) are high in omega-6 fatty acids, which can create eicosanoids, hormonelike chemicals that can lead to inflammation and blood vessel damage.	Some good, some bad
Polyunsaturated fatty acids: omega-3s	These fats lower both your HDL and your LDL. Omega-3 fatty acids are extremely beneficial and have been shown to reduce inflammation, heart disease, risk of heart attacks, and have also shown promise in helping to relieve a host of other conditions, from diabetes to bipolar disorder.	Great! The best of all fats

We need that fat to think, grow, and absorb essential vitamins and antioxidants. Fat makes foods taste good and helps us feel satisfied. Healthy fats help our hearts and feed our brains. Take a look here for your best bets—as well as what to stay away from.

Form	Sources
Monounsaturated fats are soft at room temperature but begin to harden in the fridge.	**Best Choice:** Extra virgin olive oil *Other sources:* Almonds Avocadoes Canola oil Cashews Macadamia nuts Olive oil Peanut oil Peanuts Pecans Pistachios Sesame oil
Polyunsaturated fats remain liquid at room temperature.	**Best Choice:** Walnuts *Other sources:* Corn oil Flaxseeds Margarine Mayonnaise Pumpkin seeds Safflower oil Sunflower seeds
Polyunsaturated fats remain liquid at room temperature.	**Best Choice:** Fish oil supplements* *Other sources:* Wild Pacific salmon Anchovies Cabbage Canola oil Cauliflower Cloves Flaxseeds Mackerel Oregano Soy oil Steamed broccoli Tofu Walnuts

continued on the following page

Type	Action/Benefits	Good or Bad
Saturated fats	These fats raise your LDL cholesterol, but they also elevate your HDL cholesterol. Some researchers believe that saturated fats are not nearly as dangerous as has been suggested because their effects on LDL and HDL actually cancel each other out.	Good in moderation
Trans fats: industrially produced	These fats raise LDL, lower HDL, increase inflammation, among many other bad things.	All bad, all the time
Trans fats: animal sources	The jury is still out. These fats may lower your body fat, LDL cholesterol, total cholesterol, and triglycerides. But they may also increase insulin resistance and fatty liver. What is clear is that this type of "ruminant" trans fat is not nearly as dangerous as industrially produced trans fat.	Some bad, some good

Form	Sources
Saturated fats are solid at room temperature.	**Best Choice:** Coconut oil *Other sources:* Bacon Butter Cheese Chicken Cocoa butter Cream Cream cheese Ice cream Palm kernel oil Palm oil Pork Shortening Sour cream Turkey Whole milk
Trans fats are solid at room temperature, but melt when heated.	**Best Choice:** None! *Other sources:* Baked goods Bread Breakfast cereal Cakes Candy Chips Cookies Crackers Dessert toppings Fried foods Gravy Margarine Pies Popcorn Salad dressing Shortening
Ruminant trans fats are solid at room temperature.	**Best Choice:** Organic, pasture-raised beef *Other sources:* Butter Cheese Lamb Venison Whole milk

RIGHTING THE OMEGA BALANCE

We consume about 10 times more inflammation-causing omega-6 fats (from corn, soybean, and sunflower oils, for example) than we do inflammation-reducing omega-3s. As a result, the optimal ratio between omega-3s and omega-6s—2:1 to 4:1—has been completely thrown off. We're now at 14:1 up to 25:1! This diet helps you reduce the inflammation and right that balance by Removing omega-6s on one end and Restoring omega-3s on the other end.

refined grains with added sugars, salt, fats, and chemicals, and then pocket the savings themselves.

Refined grains like white pasta, flour tortillas, white rice, and white bread are devoid of many of the healthful nutrients of grains, and have a large downside: Because they are so easy to digest, they guarantee skyrocketing blood sugar and insulin spikes. Over time, those repeated spikes lead to insulin resistance and diabetes. People who never eat whole grains have a 30 percent higher risk of diabetes than people who eat just three servings of whole grains a day.

A study in the *Journal of Clinical Nutrition* found that, compared with those who eat whole grains, people who eat refined grains have almost 40 percent higher levels of C-reactive protein, a sign of chronic, low-level inflammation in the blood vessels that's associated with heart attack and stroke. And there's no doubt that these refined grains make you fat—these "fast" carbs are so easy to eat, and so *not* filling, that we often don't wake up from our carb-coma until our fingers hit the bottom of the bag.

Corn and wheat are among the worst insulin offenders. The availability of corn flour and cereal products has almost doubled in the last thirty years, and wheat products have increased more than 20 percent. On the other hand, availability of barley, a nutritional wunderkind, has dropped by a third. In contrast with corn's meager nutritional offerings, barley packs more than thirteen grams of fiber in a single cup, helps stabilize blood sugar, and is a fantastic source of selenium, which is essential for thyroid production. It's also rich in magnesium, which helps lower triglycerides and dangerous blood lipids in diabetics. Also consider oats—in addition to their miraculous work on cholesterol, oats significantly lower blood sugar and enhance immune system function.

Can someone explain to me why the average American has access to 31 pounds of corn and 134 pounds of wheat, but only 4 pounds of oats and less than a pound of barley? Why on earth can't we get more of the grains that have actually been proven to help us?

Hormone Homework: *Go through your cabinets and fridge and get rid of any processed grain product that doesn't say "100 percent whole ___ " as the* *first ingredient. I'd love for you to get rid of all your processed grains, but if you must keep them, be sure they have at least 2 grams of fiber per serving. Beware: Products billed simply as "whole grain" are required to have only 51 percent whole grain. (Isn't that really "half grain"?)*

▶ ANTINUTRIENT #3: HIGH-FRUCTOSE CORN SYRUP

In the late seventies, the medical establishment laughed at Dr. Atkins when he said that fat didn't make people fat, carbohydrates made people fat. People thought he was nuts. He was even called in front of Congress to defend himself and his diet.

At that point, less than 15 percent of Americans were obese.

Then the low-fat dogma really kicked in, and in the decade that followed, the obesity rate shot up 8 percentage points. Now here we are thirty years later, and we're at 32 percent. The rise has been exponential. And thirty years after Atkins asserted his controversial stance, surprise, surprise, we take it as common knowledge that carbohydrates make you fat. Our bad.

This reversal of accepted wisdom won't take back those years of sugar addiction, sadly. Some of the damage was done. But we can work with our hormones to teach our bodies to react to food the way it did before we overwhelmed our insulin response systems.

The only way we'll do this is to dump the most evil refined grain of all, high-fructose corn syrup (HFCS). Get this: The U.S. production of HFCS went from 3,000 tons in 1967 to *9,227,000 tons* in 2005. Production has increased 350 percent since 1980 alone. While our average consumption of refined sugar has slowly dwindled in the past forty years, our consumption of HFCS has shot up almost twenty-fold. Tufts University researchers reported that Americans consume more calories from HFCS than from any other source.

As one of the cheapest sweeteners around, HFCS helps processed-food companies boost their profits for pennies, but all it does for us is boost our fat-storing hormones. A recent University of Florida study found that a high-fructose diet directly causes leptin resistance in lab rats. Another study, done at the University of Pennsylvania, found that fructose doesn't suppress hunger hormone ghrelin levels the way that glucose (table sugar) does. Women who ate fructose instead of glucose had higher ghrelin levels throughout the day, overnight, and into the next day.

Why does your body react this way? Well, for one thing, glucose is metabolized by all your cells; fructose must be metabolized in the liver. HFCS somehow tricks the body into not releasing insulin and leptin, two hormones your body releases when you're done eating. And unlike regular sugar, HFCS does nothing to dampen ghrelin, whose rising levels demand that your body eat more. So if you eat or drink HFCS, you'll actually continue to consume more calories, even twenty-four hours later, than you would had you just eaten plain table sugar. HFCS also increases triglycerides, and high triglycerides prevent leptin from working in the brain, so it can't tell you to stop eating.

You've probably seen ads from the Corn Refiners Association, trying to make it seem like people who avoid HFCS are paranoid. Don't buy their crap—and certainly don't eat it!

Hormone Homework: *I have a zero tolerance policy for this garbage. Train yourself to see the initials HFCS as short for "poison" and just say NO.*

ANTINUTRIENT #4: ARTIFICIAL SWEETENERS

The good news? The per capita consumption of regular soda has begun to drop by half a gallon each year. We're still at a staggering thirty-five gallons a year, from an all-time high of almost forty gallons in 1998.

The bad news? We're replacing it with diet soda—climbing steadily at almost half a gallon a year.

We think, "If sugar is bad, artificial sweeteners must be the answer, right?" Hell, no. The irony is that artificial sweeteners may put us in even greater metabolic danger than sugar or HFCS. A huge retrospective study of ninety-five hundred people over nine years found that eating meat and fried foods and drinking diet soda were the three most prominent risk factors of whether people developed metabolic syndrome. Compared with people who drank none, those who drank just one can of diet soda a day had a 34 percent greater incidence of metabolic syndrome.

Huh? How is this possible? Don't diet sodas take away the sugar?

HIDDEN HIGH-FRUCTOSE CORN SYRUP

As the most abundant source of calories and one of the cheapest ingredients in our food supply, HFCS has found its way into everything. Check labels! Make any amount of HFCS your deal breaker. (After looking at this list, you might wonder what the heck you can eat. Don't panic: Many of these foods come in healthy forms as well, such as whole grain hot dog and hamburger buns, organic yogurt without HFCS, plenty of organic lunch meats. You simply need to know where to find them and what to look for—that's what chapter 6 is all about.)

FOODS THAT COMMONLY CONTAIN HFCS
(PROCESSED, NONORGANIC VERSIONS OF THE FOLLOWING):

Applesauce	Cocktail sauce	Ketchup
Baked beans	Cola and other sodas	Lunch meat
Baking mixes	Cookies	Mayonnaise
Barbecue sauce	Cough syrup	Pasta sauce
Bread	Crackers	Peanut butter
Bread crumbs	English muffins	Pickles
Breakfast cereal	Fruit drinks	Protein bars
Candy	Fruit juice blends	Relish
Canned fruit	Hot dog and hamburger buns	Salad dressing
Cereal bars	Ice cream	
Chocolate milk	Jams and jellies	

Studies on animals give us a clue to what's happening here. Researchers at Purdue University found that when animals were fed yogurt with saccharin they later consumed more calories, gained more weight, and put on more body fat than animals that were fed yogurt sweetened with glucose, a natural sugar with the same number of calories—fifteen per teaspoon—as table sugar. The theory goes that just as we can have mental and emotional associations with certain tastes, our bodies have caloric associations with sweet tastes.

Normally, when we eat sugar, our body registers sweetness and comes to understand that very sweet things mean lots of calories. However, when we repeatedly drink diet soda, this understanding breaks down—your appetite says, "Okay, here's the sweetness, but there aren't many calories—that must mean I have to eat a lot of sweet things to get my needed calories." The next time you're given something sweet to eat, your body doesn't recognize how many calories they hold, so you overeat them. And then, in contrast to those people who ate sugar to begin with, you don't make up for those excess calories by eating less at later meals.

TOSSING ALL SUGARS

Just because HFCS is evil doesn't necessarily put a halo over other sugars' heads. No, we still have way too much of the noncorn variety in our diets as well. The average American eats more than 30 teaspoons of sugar a day—that's more than 114 pounds of sugar a year! To put it in perspective, that's about how much I weigh.

Sugar is everywhere and you want to be sure to eat it in extreme moderation. The World Health Organization recommends no more than 12 to 15 teaspoons a day, or 48 to 60 grams. I prefer that you keep it as low as possible. Check out sugar in its many aliases below. (I'll give you a hint: Anything that ends in "-ose" is a sugar.)

OTHER NAMES FOR SUGAR

Beet sugar	Glucose	Malt syrup
Brown sugar	Grape sugar	Maple syrup
Corn sweetener	High-fructose corn syrup	Molasses
Corn syrup	Honey	Raw sugar
Dextrose	Invert corn syrup	Rice syrup
Evaporated cane juice	Invert sugar	Sucrose
Fructose	Lactose	Sugar
Fruit juice concentrates	Malt	Syrup
Galactose	Maltose	

This next part is even scarier. The Purdue study also found that as the animals continued to eat the artificial sweeteners, their *metabolism* started to "forget" that most sweet things *do* have a lot of calories. Scary! So there's a good chance that when you finally do break down and have that chocolate-glazed doughnut, your body thinks, "No big deal," and doesn't bother burning up the calories because *sweetness doesn't mean anything.*

One more plausible explanation why artificial sweeteners make us fat might be the fact that aspartame, also known as NutraSweet, is an excitotoxin, a chemical that may cause permanent damage to our brain's appetite center. (See "Antinutrient #9: Glutamates" for an explanation of excitotoxin's link to obesity.) And the earlier these neural changes begin, the worse it is. A study at the University of Alberta, Canada, found that baby rats that ate more diet foods in their childhood had a greater chance of becoming obese later in life. Researchers called it "taste-conditioning process"—we might call it the "Diet Soda Backlash."

Hormone Homework: *As a recovering Diet Coke addict who would ingest Splenda by the boatloads, I feel a bit hypocritical to say "Don't eat any artificial sweeteners." This is really a case of "Please do as I say, not as I have done."*

ANTINUTRIENT #5: ARTIFICIAL PRESERVATIVES AND COLORS

Aside from the risks from HFCS and artificial sweeteners, here's one more reason to avoid soda. A major bottler settled a lawsuit with a group of parents who claimed that several of the company's products contained high levels of benzene, a known carcinogen also linked to serious thyroid damage. Benzoate salts are added to soda to prevent mold growth. A *Consumer Reports* test found that when drinks with these salts sit in plastic soda bottles in direct sunlight or in heat, dangerous levels of benzene can form. Coca-Cola removed the additives from several of their products, but these preservatives—and many others that have not been adequately tested—remain in many other sodas on the shelf.

Hormone Homework: *Don't take any chances—avoid any soda with sodium benzoate or potassium benzoate and vitamin C (ascorbic acid), as the combination of these two additives can create the benzene. If you must drink it, be sure to store your soda in a cool, dark place.*

How could an idea with such a good intention—to prevent spoilage and food poisoning—go so incredibly wrong? The artificial preservatives in our food supply age us and create all kinds of autoimmune diseases, from multiple forms of cancer to MS. Researchers are discovering more and more that these preservatives are also likely to destroy our biochemistry, inhibit our metabolism, and interfere with our ability to lose weight.

Let's take one example: A common preservative, butylated hydroxyanisole, or BHA, has been "generally recognized as safe" by the FDA, but is still "reasonably anticipated to be a human carcinogen." (How much sense does that make?) This chemical antioxidant helps prevent food spoilage, but it's also an endocrine disruptor. One study determined that the more BHA a male rat received, the less testosterone and T4 he had circulating in his body. These little guys stopped wanting sex, they had fewer and weaker sperm, and their testes shrunk. Plus, their livers and adrenal glands swelled up and their thyroid glands were completely screwed.

Now consider that we eat BHA in hundreds of foods, including butter, lard, cereals, baked goods, sweets, beer, vegetable oils, potato chips, snack foods, nuts, dehydrated potatoes, flavoring agents, sausage, poultry and meat products, dry mixes for beverages and desserts, glazed fruits, chewing gum, active dry yeast, defoaming agents for beet sugar and yeast, and emulsion stabilizers for shortening. BHA is also found in food packaging, lipsticks, lip glosses, mascaras, eye shadows, and facial creams. Even if the individual levels of BHA are "generally recognized as safe," what happens when we use multiple products that all include them, or eat multiple servings? And consider this: BHA could be replaced by vitamin E or left out of some foods altogether. So why take the risk?

Hormone Homework: *Check packages for signs of BHA, which also goes by the names anisole, butylated hydroxy-; antioxyne B; antrancine 12; butylhydroxyanisole; tert-butyl hydroxyanisole; embanox; nepantiox 1-F; phenol, tert-butyl-4-methoxy; phenol, (1,1-dimethylethyl)-4-methoxy-; sustane 1-F; tenox BHA. (You're probably looking at this list thinking, "Are you kidding me? How am I going to remember any of those?" That's exactly my point— see how it might be easier just to stay away from processed foods altogether?)*

We could have this same conversation about so many chemical additives, for so many devastating health risks. The debate has raged for decades about the link between kids' behavior problems and artificial coloring and preservatives. Pediatricians have often pooh-poohed parents' concerns about these chemicals, citing government "generally regarded as safe" guidelines and saying that parents are just looking for scapegoats for their kids' bad behavior. But a recent randomized, double-blind, placebo-controlled study—in other words, rock-solid research—in *The Lancet* proved otherwise. After preschoolers and grade-school kids ate an additive-free diet for six weeks, then reintroduced additives into their diets, their hyperactivity levels rose dramatically. Considering that the prevalence of ADHD in this country has risen to almost one in ten kids, and a bunch of them are being put on medication at as young as four, maybe we should do something about this!

Hormone Homework: *Always choose foods with the least number of artificial chemicals for your kids, and be on the lookout for artificial colors, many of which have been linked with thyroid, adrenal, bladder, kidney, and brain cancer. The worst offenders are blue 1 and 2, green 3, red 3, and yellow 6. But really, why subject them to any of this crap? Choose color-free medication, and when you allow them a treat, make sure it's a small portion of the real thing. For example, give them real ice cream instead of rainbow freezy pops.*

PLAYING THE ODDS ON FOOD ADDITIVES

Food additives are evil. But sometimes they are a necessary evil. (Really, who wants to get a nice case of botulism?) The trick is to know which is the lesser of two evils.

Safe	(Sometimes) Necessary Evil	Downright Evil
Safe or may even have health benefits	Risks are minor, but keep consumption down	Avoid at all costs
Alpha tocopherol (aka vitamin E)	Carageenan	Aspartame, saccharin, sucralose
Ascorbic acid (aka vitamin C)	Gelatin	Butylated hydroxyanisole (BHA)
Citric acid, sodium citrate	Lecithin	Monosodium glutamate (MSG)
Beta-carotene (aka precursor to vitamin A)	Maltodextrin	Olestra
Inulin	Mono- and diglycerides	Partially hydrogenated vegetable oil
Lactic acid	Phosphates, phosphoric acid	Potassium bromate
Oligofructose	Oat fiber, wheat fiber	Sodium benzoate, benzoic acid
Phytosterols or phytostanols	Sorbic acid, potassium sorbate	Sodium nitrate, sodium nitrite
Thiamin mononitrate (aka Vitamin B_1)	Vanillin, ethyl vanillin	Sulfites (sodium bisulfite, sodium Dioxide)

Source: Center for Science in the Public Interest (www.cspinet.org/reports/chemcuisine.htm)

Some of the absolute worst preservatives for your metabolism are used in processed meats. A landmark NIH study of more than nine thousand people found that the single greatest predictor of a person's chance of developing metabolic syndrome was a steady diet of hamburgers, hot dogs, and processed meats. The sodium nitrate and nitrite in bacon, ham, lunch meat, and hot dogs give processed meat its pink color and prevent the spread of bacteria. But much of that preventive protection could easily be achieved with adequate refrigeration without risks to our health. After analyzing more than seven thousand studies on diet and cancer risk, the American Institute for Cancer Research estimated that for every 3.5 ounces of processed meat you eat per day—the equivalent of one hot dog and two slices of smoked turkey breast—your risk of colon cancer shoots up by 42 percent.

Hormone Homework: *Avoid any processed meats, especially those that include nitrates or nitrites. (Ask the deli counter clerk to read the label on the meat before slicing it for you.) Choose fresh meat—look for organic or, at* *the very least, nitrite-free meats. More and more grocery-store chains are developing their own low-cost brands.*

▶ ANTINUTRIENT #6: GLUTAMATES

Now we move on to our pal glutamates, most frequently talked about as monosodium glutamate, or MSG. Many people mistakenly think MSG is a preservative. Were that the case, it might actually have a semiplausible excuse for being in food. No, glutamates are "flavor enhancers."

Glutamates do exist in natural foods like cheese and meat. But the low levels of "bound" glutamates in natural foods are nowhere near the levels of "free" glutamates currently being exploited by the processed-foods industry. You've chowed on MSG in everything from canned raviolis, soup, and canned tuna to bouillon, ice cream, and ranch dressing. A recent *New York Times* article noted that Doritos have *five kinds* of glutamates.

Glutamates are produced by hydrolyzing proteins, a process that "frees" the glutamates from the protein. When added to foods, glutamates enhance the savory taste experience—indeed, we probably have taste receptors for glutamates just like we have taste receptors for salty, sweet, bitter, and sour tastes. Sounds good, right? But it turns out that high levels of free glutamates also mess with your brain chemistry, big-time.

Glutamates are a form of excitotoxin, which studies as far back as the 1950s have shown to be devastating to the nervous system. Excitotoxins dive into the brain with relative ease, excite brain cells, and can rapidly cause permanent brain damage and eventual cell death. One area of the brain particularly vulnerable to excess glutamates is the hypothalamus, ground zero for hunger hormones like neuropeptide Y.

Although the debate about MSG's safety remains heated, some researchers assert that animals fed MSG sustained damage to their hypothalamus that led to obesity and endocrine problems later in life. One possible reason is that MSG damages your leptin receptors, causing your body to produce more, while simultaneously creating leptin resistance in the brain.

The worst part? Some processed foods not only have one form of glutamate, they may have two, three, or even *four* kinds. (See "The Glutamate Finder" that follows.) As with all of these scary chemicals, who's to

THE GLUTAMATE FINDER

The government has decreed that anything that has monosodium glutamate in it must say "Contains MSG." Does that mean that if your food doesn't have the label, it doesn't have glutamates? Absolutely not—it just doesn't have that particular glutamate.

Don't be fooled by the words "natural flavor" or "spices" either. Foods with natural flavors or spices could, in fact, be jam-packed with glutamates, and you'd never know it! Check out this list of code words for hidden free glutamic acids in your processed foods:

LIKELY SOURCES OF MSG

Autolyzed yeast	Monosodium glutamate
Calcium caseinate	Natrium glutamate (*natrium* is Latin/German
Gelatin	for "sodium")
Glutamate	Sodium caseinate
Glutamic acid	Textured protein
Hydrolyzed corn gluten	Yeast extract
Hydrolyzed protein (wheat, milk, soy, whey—	Yeast food
any protein that is hydrolyzed)	Yeast nutrient
Monopotassium glutamate	

say what their synergistic effects could be? By padding their foods with several varieties of glutamates, food companies want you to *love* their food, so you'll keep coming back for more. This is your brain on corn chips. Just say no!

Hormone Homework: *As you eliminate as many glutamates as possible from your diet, also explore ways to boost the natural flavor of foods. Fermented foods, wine, soy sauce, Parmesan cheese, anchovies, and ketchup are all naturally flavorful. Also, roasting, smoking, or slow grilling makes foods taste rich and savory. And seek out the organic versions and enjoy without fear!*

▶ LESS-THAN-STELLAR FOODS

While whether to eat some of these foods is a black-and-white issue—may another gram of hydrogenated fat *never* pass your lips, for example—some foods are okay in smaller quantities. Let's take a look at some less-than-stellar options in our food supply, and set an upper limit to how much you should have. Your hormone levels may be fine with small quantities, but they may become overwhelmed with more.

LESS-THAN-STELLAR OPTION #1: STARCHY ROOT VEGETABLES

You'll find out how much I love vegetables in chapter 6. But one type is not on the top of my list: starchy vegetables.

Just as we store our energy as glycogen, plants store their energy as starch. As such, starchy vegetables are more calorie-dense than non-starchy vegetables. Nonstarchy vegetables, like broccoli, spinach, and green peppers, have 25 calories and 5 grams of carbs per half cup cooked serving, and they cause a negligible bump in your blood sugar. Starchy carbs, on the other hand, have 80 calories and 15 grams of carbs per half cup cooked serving—and most have an immediate and dramatic impact on your blood sugar and insulin. And which vegetable could you imagine yourself overindulging in, potatoes or spinach?

Root vegetables and other starchy vegetables, such as potatoes, beets, corn, and peas, have some redeeming nutritional qualities—potatoes are a fantastic source of potassium, for example—but they're missing out on a lot of the more potent antioxidants and other phytochemicals that are more prevalent in nonstarchy vegetables. When you put those two things together—more calories and less nutrition—I think you know where I stand on the matter.

Hormone Homework: *Aim for less than two servings of starchy vegetables a day. If you're going to have them, try interesting types like parsnips, a proven cancer fighter, or beets, full of folate to help lower levels of heart-attack-inducing homocysteine in the blood. I'm also a fan of sweet potatoes, packed with free-radical-fighting beta-carotene and vitamin C. Anything but the usual suspects of corn, peas, and potatoes—God knows you don't need more corn!*

LESS-THAN-STELLAR OPTION #2: TROPICAL, DRIED, AND CANNED FRUITS

Watermelon, pineapple, banana, mango—basically all tropical fruits—are high in sugar and should be consumed in limited quantities. But when I say "limited," I mean five servings a *week* (about one a day is okay). Dried and other processed fruits should be treated as processed foods—i.e., not good for you—so let them be. Many dried fruits use preservatives called sulfites, which can, in some people, cause severe allergic reactions such as hives, nausea, diarrhea, shortness of breath, or even fatal shock. Not good. Even grapes can be packed with sulfites when they're shipped.

Canned fruits, even when packed in their own juices, are considerably higher in sugar than when you just eat them off the tree or vine. And heavy syrups—well, 'nuff said on that front. That's just like grabbing a cup of corn syrup and dunking in a forkful of fruit. So gross.

Hormone Homework: *One dried fruit you might want to slip into rotation? Dried plums, aka prunes. A good source of both soluble and insoluble fiber, dried plums are excellent for your digestion and help manage your blood sugar at the same time. Just watch your portions—each individual prune is twenty-five calories.*

LESS-THAN-STELLAR OPTION #3: EXCESS SOY

For years, we heard about what a super food soy was—this lean protein helped lower cholesterol, protect bones, improve circulation, reduce inflammation, and lower the risks of cancer and diabetes. Soy was going to save the universe, from the sound of things.

The food industry's inevitable reaction? If a bit of something is good (and cheap!), way, way more of it must be better. Almost overnight, every processed-food product seemed to have added soy or isoflavones, the flavonoid in soy that showed promise in many of these health claims. Premenopausal women were promised freedom from hot flashes with soy supplements; heart patients were chowing down on huge bags of soy nuts.

There's only one problem: Isoflavones are endocrine disruptors that mimic the actions of estrogen. When we get isoflavones from natural products, we're fine—the body knows what to do with the 38 grams of isoflavones in a half cup of tofu. But it's really not sure what to do with the 160 grams of concentrated isoflavones in a Revival soy bar.

While at first isoflavones were hailed as a shield against breast cancer, a growing body of research suggests that isoflavones might be dangerous for women who are either postmenopausal or at risk for breast cancer. The estrogenlike activity of isoflavones encourages abnormal cell growth in those already at risk. When you consider how many processed foods use soy as a cheap protein source, and you add in the rising tide of environmental estrogens, you can see that the last thing we need is *extra* estrogen supplementation!

Plus, many soy products are made from genetically modified (GMO) soybeans. In fact, 85 percent of all soybeans planted in the United States are GMO. Given that we suspect GMOs threaten biodiversity and the long-term health of our farmland, but we know *nothing* about their long-term health effects, I'd rather we just stay away from them.

A little bit of soy can be a good thing—it's rich in lean protein, omega-3s, iron, magnesium, and various cancer fighters such as saponins and phytosterols. And some of the phytoestrogen activity can be protective, especially for younger women. But given the problems soy can create for those with thyroid issues (soy is a known goitrogen) and those at risk of breast cancer (you can put most American women in that category), I recommend you limit your soy intake to whole foods that have the content of isoflavones nature intended them to have, and eat only two servings *per week*.

Hormone Homework: *I'm all for a few chunks of tofu or tempeh in a stir-fry, and miso soup is also acceptable—these more natural uses of fermented soy have been around forever and may be part of why Japanese women have a lower incidence of breast cancer. But steer clear of processed products with isolated soy proteins and/or high levels of isoflavones, like soy nuts, soy-fortified bars and drinks, soy flour, soy cheese, soy milk, and faux meats. And if you're a parent, really do your homework before you put your baby on soy formula. Those tiny bodies are getting such concentrated doses of estrogens that some are growing breasts! Soy formula can damage babies' immune systems and has been linked with a 90 percent higher usage of allergy and asthma medications later in life. Beware.*

▶ LESS-THAN-STELLAR OPTION #4: EXCESS ALCOHOL

You've probably heard a lot lately about wine. "It extends your life! Fights diabetes and heart disease! Prevents cognitive decline!" All due to the miraculous effects of resveratrol, a powerful phytochemical that fights viruses and inflammation. But there's just one thing about the amazing resveratrol—it's also a phytoestrogen.

Alcohol releases estrogen into your bloodstream, promotes fat storage, and decreases muscle growth. As soon as you have a drink, your body gobbles up all the glycogen in your liver, makes you hungry, and reduces your inhibitions, so you're more likely to grab that chicken wing or stuffed potato skin at happy hour. You also burn way less fat, and burn it more slowly, than normal—*Prevention* magazine estimates that just two drinks can cut your fat-burning ability by 73 percent.

While some argue that resveratrol's phytoestrogen nature is actually protective against cancer, alcohol itself is a breast cancer risk. One study found that alcohol helps develop the most common type of breast cancer tumors, those with both estrogen and progesterone receptors. Analyzing data from more than 184,000 women, scientists deduced that one to two drinks a day increases your risk of developing these kinds of malignant tumors by 32 percent; three or more bumps that number to 51 percent.

On the other hand, especially if you're a guy, we can't deny that wine has its benefits: it protects your heart, helps lower inflammation, fights viruses, and might even lower blood sugar in diabetics. Recently, researchers at the UC San Diego School of Medicine found that one glass of wine a day may decrease the risk, by almost 40 percent, of nonalcoholic fatty liver disease, a condition associated with insulin resistance and heart disease. Bottom line, one drink a day probably maxes out your benefits, so keep a cork in your alcohol consumption.

Hormone Homework: *If you're going to have alcohol, drink wine. (See "Get Your Drink On, Organically" above.) Women who had an occasional glass of wine (one or fewer per day) increased their breast cancer risk by only 7 percent, which might net out with other health benefits—provided you don't have other individual breast cancer risks. Ask your doctor to help you assess your personal risk of breast cancer.*

GET YOUR DRINK ON, ORGANICALLY

Organic wines are produced without pesticides or preservatives, such as sulfites. About 1 in 20 people are allergic to sulfites, and people with asthma are particularly vulnerable. Many swear sulfites are behind that "cheap wine" hangover.

All wine contains sulfites, but added sulfites can be 10 to 20 times the natural amount. Red wines don't even need 'em; rosé and white wines have more; and sweet wines, the most. Check for added sulfites on the label. Once you've started drinking wines without sulfites, you'll never want to go back—you'll taste the difference right away.

LESS-THAN-STELLAR OPTION #5:
FULL-FAT DAIRY AND FATTY MEATS

Fats are no longer the dietetic demons they once were. We know that some fats are incredibly healthy for you, such as omega-3s, found in flaxseed and wild-caught salmon; and conjugated linoleic acids (CLA), found in the meat and milk of organic pasture-fed cows. But that doesn't necessarily mean all "full" fats and dairy are good. Sure, saturated fats are not the best when you're trying to reduce your risks of heart disease. And while some hard-core Atkins types argue that saturated fats help you lose weight, we have a ways to go before the science proves that beyond a doubt. There are conflicting arguments and convincing cases on both sides, but the biggest danger of full-fat meat and dairy is their tremendous endocrine-disrupting power from the garbage that is put in them.

Eating animal products is the number-one way we absorb dioxins—livestock absorbs industrial pollution from incinerators. All the pesticides, hormones, and other chemicals used in industrial farming—whether to increase meat growth, boost milk production, or kill bugs and fungus on crops—find their way into nonorganic meat and dairy. And stay there. Many chemicals used in farming "bioaccumulate," or collect, in the animal's fat tissue. And as soon as you consume that flesh, those toxins take up residence in your fatty tissue and camp out for decades. *Consumer Reports* cites an EPA estimate that you are ten times more likely to develop cancer from dioxin—with about a one in one hundred chance—if you eat a high-fat diet, precisely because of the high levels of this toxin in meat and dairy.

The sad thing is that even organic meats have some trace of pesticides and chemicals, just like every human born every second in this country. The result: Your body is like a giant toxic-waste dump, collecting all the chemical crap in the food supply—and holding on to it.

Before we get all bummed out here, let's get back to the basics of weight control. The primary reason not to eat full-fat dairy and meat when trying to lose pounds comes down to simple math: Ounce for ounce, those foods have way more calories than leaner and lower-fat options.

Hormone Homework: *Always go organic for meat and dairy. Also, try to get the lowest fat content possible—choose leaner cuts of meat (look for the words* loin *or* round, *such as "sirloin" and "eye of round"), trim any visible*

PREPARE FOOD TO MINIMIZE TOXINS

Removing certain foods is only half the picture—you also have to prepare foods in ways that minimize the chance that endocrine disruptors will leak into your food. Here are 20 tips to help you do just that:

1. Remove visible fat and skin from any chicken, meat, or fish.
2. Don't eat nonorganic full-fat animal products; choose skim or 1 percent dairy whenever possible.
3. Peel skins to eliminate pesticide residue from vegetables and fruits.
4. Remove the outer layers of cabbage and lettuce and throw them away.
5. Chop off the tops of fruits such as apples and pears to avoid pesticides that might drain into the stem area.
6. Wash reusable plastic drinking bottles by hand, never in the dishwasher. If they get cracked or cloudy, recycle them and get a stainless steel bottle for water.
7. Grill, bake, or broil meats. Don't fry them.
8. Avoid "everything but the kitchen sink" meat products, such as hot dogs, bologna, and sausage—even minimize organic versions as they, too, will have concentrated toxins in their organs.
9. Wash fruits and veggies with gentle dish soap that doesn't contain scents or phosphates.
10. Don't store food in plastic containers. Throw them out and replace them with glass ones.
11. Stay away from cans as much as possible by eating seasonal produce.
12. Buy canned foods from Eden Foods because they don't use BPA in their organic bean cans.
13. Buy broth, juice, milk, and other liquid products in cardboard containers instead of cans.
14. Don't use plastic wrap; if you must, choose BPA-free Saran.
15. Never microwave with plastic wrap or other plastic containers; if you need to cover a dish, use a chlorine-free paper towel or another inverted dish as a top.
16. Don't buy boil-in-bag or microwave-in-bag vegetables or rice.
17. When grilling, use leaner cuts of meat or fish that won't create fat-drip flare-ups. These flare-ups deposit known carcinogens, called heterocyclic amines (HCAs) or polycyclic aromatic hydrocarbons (PAHs), on meat. (Grilled veggies and fruit don't have them.)
18. Throw away any juices that drip from grilled meat, fish, or chicken.
19. Use glass baby bottles or bottles with liners.
20. Buy your veggies, fruits, meat, and dairy from your local organic farmers market as often as possible!

fat, and choose skim or 1 percent dairy products. Try to get the majority of your fats from unsaturated and omega-3 fats as often you can.

> ## LESS-THAN-STELLAR OPTION #6: CANNED FOODS

We get almost 20 percent of our food from cans. Where do we live, in a fallout shelter?

Look, I'm a realist. I know that when you're busy, it's much better for you to whip open a can of Trader Joe's chili and nuke it than it is to cruise to the Wendy's drive-through. I get it. But I still want you to get away from eating vegetables from cans instead of from a farmers market. They're not the same.

First of all, you're not getting nearly the nutritional bang for your caloric buck. Many veggies lose up to 90 percent of their original nutrition power in the canning process. Second, canned foods are typically very high in sodium—some cans of soup have 2,000 milligrams!

But perhaps worst is that cans are lined with plastic that contains BPA. The Environmental Working Group did a study and found that for 1 in 10 cans of regular food—and 1 in 3 cans of baby formula—a single serving was 200 times the FDA's maximum safe level for other industrial chemicals. The problem is, our government doesn't currently *have* a safety standard when it comes to BPA in cans—the sky's the limit, folks! A study in the United Kingdom found that out of 62 cans purchased in supermarkets there, 40 tested positive for BPA. As you'll recall from chapter 3, BPA is linked to insulin resistance, early puberty, prostate cancer, and a host of other lovely conditions caused by hormone disruption.

Hormone Homework: *This is reason #794 to stay away from processed foods. If you must eat out of cans, buy organic, low-salt options. Try to minimize your exposure to BPA as much as possible. Canned soup, pasta, and baby formula have the most. As of press time, Eden organic beans (www.edenfoods. com) was the only brand packed in a special can with a natural resin-based liner that doesn't include BPA. Almost every other can in America (with the exception of some canned fruit) has BPA in its lining—and, thus, in your food.*

▶ LESS-THAN-STELLAR OPTION #7: CAFFEINE

We've come to my Achilles' heel—and I think I'm not alone. More than half of us drink three to four cups of coffee every day. Maybe you do it for energy, maybe because you've heard that some studies show caffeine enhances your workout performance and helps to burn fat. But don't chug that pot of coffee just yet.

It's true that pure caffeine in moderate doses (200 to 400 milligrams a day) can elevate metabolism by up to 6 percent, improve cognitive function, and even inhibit insulin resistance.

Here's the catch. Nonorganic coffee (or Red Bull or Diet Coke) isn't going to give you any fat-burning effect. Those studies were done using isolated caffeine as a supplement, paired with other specific substances, in a tightly controlled lab setting. It doesn't apply to caffeine paired with excitotoxins or sugar or milk solids or whatever else is lurking in your cup or can.

Even worse, when caffeine is abused, it damages your metabolism and hormone balance. Caffeine stimulates your central nervous system, which makes your endocrine system think that you are threatened in some way. With that third cup of coffee at your desk each day, you kick your body into fight-or-flight mode while you're just checking e-mail. Your adrenals pump out epinephrine and norepinephrine. These two stress hormones set into motion a cascade of fattening hormonal actions: Your liver releases blood sugar for quick energy, your pancreas spits out insulin to counter the sugar, your blood sugar dips because of the insulin's actions. Also, your blood vessels constrict, making you feel like your blood sugar is dipping even further, so you head for the vending machine. Ever notice how you crave something sweet somewhere between the first and second cup of coffee? That's your body reacting to this sudden feeling of blood sugar shortage.

The acids in one cup of coffee will elevate your cortisol for up to fourteen hours. Now, if you sip caffeinated drinks all day, you switch on your stress reaction over and over—your short-term energy burns out, you grab another cup, repeat the hormonal cycle again, and effectively turn yourself into an addict.

Caffeine abuse overstimulates and eventually wears down your adrenals; it also inflicts the long-term effects of real stress in your body: Oxygen flow to your brain slows, your immune system is suppressed, the excess cortisol increases your appetite and encourages fat to pack on your belly, and, last, your continued insulin spikes help to create insulin resistance.

To make matters worse, when it's time to restore yourself with rest, the caffeine you drank during the daytime may prevent you from getting adequate sleep that night—and you now know that lack of sleep itself creates insulin resistance.

The phosphoric acid in colas and coffee interferes with your calcium absorption. In addition to being brutal on your bones, this calcium deficiency—and the caffeine itself—can make the symptoms of PMS much worse, including increased breast tenderness, irritability, and nervousness.

The National Academy of Sciences released a report claiming that caffeinated beverages can be calculated in your daily water intake—but if you ask me, that's bogus. Caffeine is a diuretic, draining precious water from your body at the very moment you're trying to flush out the toxins. When you're dehydrated, your blood volume decreases, reducing the amount of oxygen that can get to your muscles, making them less effective at burning fat. There's no debate here: Get your water from *water*.

Hormone Homework: *Take this opportunity to transition to green tea. You'll still get a caffeine boost, but green tea has been shown to promote fat oxidation at rest and is believed to prevent obesity and improve insulin sensitivity. Green tea also reduces the risk of breast and prostate cancer. But guys, take note: Part of the reason green tea works is by lowering the amount of circulating sex hormones in the body. In other words, while it helps reduce dangerous levels of estrogen, it also lowers testosterone—so tread lightly. No more than one cup a day.*

Limit yourself to one to two caffeinated beverages a day, and drink one extra glass of water for every caffeinated beverage you drink. Make sure you finish drinking both of them by noon. I want that caffeine completely out of your system by nightfall.

NOW, THE GOOD STUFF

You've taken the first step and eliminated the foods and other products that stand in the way of your normal hormonal function. Now we're going to talk about how to choose the foods that will optimize those hormones, and get your metabolism working harder and burning higher than it has for a long time. In chapter 6, you're going to revel in all the delicious foods you *add* to your diet. On my website, you can get tons of recipes and personal meal plans that incorporate these great foods. Like I've said before, I want you to eat. But I want you to eat foods that work for you, not against you.

STEP 2—RESTORE

DISCOVER THE POWER NUTRIENTS THAT
FEED YOUR FAT-BURNING HORMONES

Now that we've Removed the antinutrients that spur your hormones to store fat, we can focus on Restoring the foods that trigger your fat-loss hormones. The main focus of Step 2 is the ten Power Nutrient Food Groups that repair your metabolism and re-create your natural hormonal equilibrium. You'll learn to eat whole, natural, real foods that help build muscle tissue and repair cells. You'll also learn about specific foods and eating habits that help support your glands and hormone production, turning on the hormones you want, and turning off those that sabotage your weight-loss efforts.

Most of all, I wanted to create a food plan that's sustainable. You may not be able to stick a bag in the microwave and call it dinner, but I've tried to make it as easy as possible to follow this diet. You might have to work a little, but the benefits are unbeatable.

> ## THE *MASTER YOUR METABOLISM* POWER NUTRIENTS

You know how much I love to go on about the power of choice. What if I told you that you have the power to reduce your risk of all obesity-related diseases, such as heart disease, cancer, diabetes, and stroke, by

1. Legumes
2. Alliums
3. Berries
4. Meat and eggs
5. Colorful fruits and veggies
6. Cruciferous veggies
7. Dark-green leafy veggies
8. Nuts and seeds
9. Organic dairy
10. Whole grains

50 percent? This life-or-death choice is made by you when you choose the foods you are going to put in your body.

Do you realize that there is nothing in our genes that tells us when to die? There are genetic codes that tell us how to grow, how to breathe, and how to sleep, but NOTHING that tells us to die. So why do we? Because we literally rust and decay our bodies from the inside out with poor food and lifestyle choices.

God/nature/whatever name you want to call it has provided us with all we need to heal ourselves. Hippocrates said, "Let food be your medicine," and boy, was he right! Some foods heal with absolutely no negative side effects, are 100 percent natural, and are as far away as your local market. I call them Power Nutrients. A Power Nutrient is a food that can dramatically improve the quality and duration of your life. These foods have been scientifically proven to help prevent and, in some cases, reverse disease. They also stabilize your hormones and rev up your metabolism—a welcome side effect you'll never get from drugs.

Following is a list of ten Power Nutrient food groups that you should consume as often as possible—I mean it! Let's look at what each one does for your body and how each helps you restore your body's metabolism. As you read about the Power Nutrients, you'll also encounter "Hormone Trigger Foods" sidebars, collections of foods that have been found to either trigger or dampen specific hormones. All the hormone-positive foods have been incorporated into this diet's food lists, meal plans, and recipes. (For handy lists of Power Nutrient foods, please see "The Master Shopping List," page 236.)

POWER NUTRIENT FOOD GROUP #1: LEGUMES

Beans and other legumes (BEST CHOICE: red beans) do have carbs, but the best kinds. For example, beans are one of the richest sources of soluble fiber, which is key to good blood sugar control. They also have resistant starch RS1, which "resists" being digested in the small intestine until it can pass into the large intestine. There, the resistant starch ferments, rebuilds the intestinal lining, and creates short-chain fatty acids, which fight systemic inflammation, cancer, and "bad" bugs in the gut, like *E. coli* and candida. Resistant starch also helps lower insulin levels, probably because it takes so long to digest that it slows down the release of blood sugar. One study found that by adding 5 percent resistant starch to your meal, you increase your postmeal fat burn—and 80 percent of that fat comes from your belly and hips, 20 percent from the fat in your meal. Gotta love that! Plus, when you eat the resistant starch in beans, you feel fuller, store less fat, lower your cholesterol and triglycerides, and improve your whole body's insulin sensitivity.

Many beans contain phytoestrogens, but unlike isoflavone-enriched processed soy products, these phytoestrogens are shown to *reduce* levels of circulating estrogen. Beans are also high in zinc and B vitamins, both proven testosterone boosters.

Hormone Homework: *Have 1 to 3 servings per day.*
- Dried beans are better than canned; soak them for six to eight hours, or overnight, in room temperature water, then drain before cooking.
- Don't avoid canned beans if that convenience encourages you to eat more legumes— the numerous health benefits of beans and lentils vastly outweigh the potential dangers of cans. (Don't forget that Eden Foods has BPA-free cans.)
- Look for no-salt varieties and rinse them thoroughly before cooking.
- No, refried beans with lard do not count! If you love that taste, look for refrieds that contain beans, salt, and water. (See the Resources on page 243 for my favorite brands.)

POWER NUTRIENT FOOD GROUP #2: THE ALLIUM FAMILY

Garlic (BEST CHOICE) and the other alliums—onions, leeks, chives, shallots, and scallions—are incredible body detoxers. They stimulate the body to produce glutathione, an antioxidant that lives within each cell, ready to fight free radicals where they live throughout the body. Glutathione's action is especially important in the liver, where it helps to remove pharmaceuticals and other endocrine-disrupting chemicals.

A certain type of flavonoids in onions, called anthocyanins, are incredible free-radical destroyers, and emerging science suggests they may also help fight obesity and diabetes. Garlic and its siblings also help to lower total cholesterol—but raise HDL—by decreasing the liver's synthesis

HORMONE TRIGGER FOODS: ESTROGEN AND PROGESTERONE

Foods that impact your estrogen levels can be a dicey business. Foods that are high in phytoestrogens may help women manage some of the less comfortable symptoms of perimenopause, such as hot flashes. But once women hit menopause, or if they have any risk of breast or uterine cancer, these extra estrogens may be risky. Ditto for guys—some phytoestrogens can help protect your heart; too many may suppress your testosterone and increase your risk of prostate cancer. They're not the only foods that can alter your estrogen balance, however. Take a look:

Estrogen Reducers	Why	Sources and Solutions
Dietary fiber	Estrogen is normally pulled from the bloodstream by the liver, which sends it through a small tube, called the bile duct, into the intestinal tract. There, fiber soaks it up like a sponge and carries it out with other waste. The more fiber there is in the diet, the better the natural "estrogen disposal system" works.	Fruits, vegetables, and whole grains, especially those high in soluble fiber, such as apples, barley, beans, psyllium, lentils, and oat bran
Flavones	May prevent adrenal hormones, such as testosterone, from being converted into estrogen	Onions, black and green tea, and apples are among the best sources of flavonol and flavones.
Green tea	A study found that green tea lowered levels of less healthy estrone while black tea raised them.	Green tea in all forms—loose, tea bags, iced tea
Indole-3-carbinol	This antioxidant helps stimulate detoxifying enzymes. Indole-3-blocks estrogen receptors on cell membranes, reducing the risk of breast and cervical cancers.	Cruciferous veggies like broccoli, cabbage, kale, and Brussels sprouts
Pomegranate	One lab study found that pomegranate juice, extract, and oil were able to block estrogenic activity by up to 80 percent and prevent several different types of breast cancer cells from multiplying. Another study found a similar effect on prostate cancer cells.	POM juice is a great source. Also try to incorporate pomegranate seeds into your salads and desserts. Their tartness adds a delicious counterpart to vanilla yogurt.

Estrogen Raisers	Why	Sources and Solutions
Alcohol	One study found that, after four weeks, postmenopausal women who had 1 drink a day increased their estrone levels by almost 7 percent. Those who had 2 drinks a day increased their estrone by 22 percent.	Stick to 1 drink a day, max. If you're at any risk for breast cancer, skip the drink altogether.
Caffeine	A study found that 2 or more cups of coffee or 4 cans of soda a day brought up levels of estrone.	Limit yourself to 1 or 2 cups max of coffee—and try to cut out soda altogether.
Fat	One Japanese study found that among lean women, dietary fat did raise estrogen levels, but the mechanism is unclear. Trans fats encourage visceral fat, which encourages extra estrone production.	Avoid any chips, crackers, cookies, or fried foods prepared with partially hydrogenated oils—they're all loaded with trans fats.
Flaxseed	Flaxseed is the richest source of secoisolariciresinol diglycoside (SDG), which is turned into lignans in the body. Similar to those in lignans are phytoestrogens that can both support healthy estrogen levels and also decrease circulating levels of estrogen by competing for receptor space. (Again, speak to your doctor about any cancer concerns.)	Buy flaxseed, grind up a little at a time, and store in the refrigerator. Add to cereal, yogurt, and smoothies. Flaxseed is also a good source of the omega-3 fatty acid ALA.
Hops	The female flowers of hops are used to make beer and contain a phytoestrogen that has been shown to reduce hot flashes.	Beer doesn't contain enough hops to make a difference—unless you drink way too much of it! But alcohol will raise estrogen levels in the blood, so hold yourself to 1 glass of beer.

continued on the following page

Estrogen Raisers	Why	Sources and Solutions
Red clover	Contains naturally occurring phytoestrogens, as well as metabolism helpers calcium, chromium, and magnesium	Most often found in supplement form, but you can also get red clover in bean sprouts.
Soy	Soy contains phytoestrogens called isoflavones. These compounds mimic estrogen, so technically they increase them. But natural soy products contain a weaker form of estrogen that blocks the receptors of stronger forms (such as estrone), so they also decrease circulating levels of estrogen. They also don't accumulate in the body and are quickly metabolized. In men and premenopausal women with no other risk factors, soy and other phytoestrogens may help reduce the risk of prostate, breast, and uterine cancers. However, if you're already at higher risk for any of those conditions, additional estrogen may raise your risk. This is why I always recommend soy in moderation. (Talk to your doctor about your personal risk of cancer as it relates to excess estrogen.)	Fermented soy products such as tofu, miso, tempeh, edamame. (Steer clear of concentrated isoflavone products, such as soy milk, soy nuts, or soy flour.) Other sources of phytoestrogens include fennel, anise, and sesame seeds.
Yams	Unclear, but somehow yams seem to decrease the metabolism of estrogen that leads to elevated levels. One study found that eating yams twice a day for a month raised estrone levels.	To be honest, to get any hormonal effects, we're talking some serious yams here—at least 2 or more a day.

of cholesterol. (Two cloves of garlic a day might be as potent as some cholesterol-lowering drugs.) Although studies in rats suggest that garlic's allicin may enhance testosterone levels, it's a little early to know. But garlic already does so much—if they prove it does increase testosterone, so much the better.

Leeks are especially cool. They take the best aspects of garlic and onions—especially manganese, a blood sugar stabilizer—and combine them with fiber, turning them into an all-around fantastic choice to keep insulin levels stable.

Hormone Homework: *Have at least 1 serving per day.*
- Crushing, chopping, or chewing garlic helps release allinase enzymes, which trigger many of its beneficial actions. At least chop the top off before you roast it—that will allow for some enzyme activity.
- Before you cook with chopped or crushed garlic, let it stand for 10 minutes to let the enzymes activate all of the beneficial compounds.
- If you can hack it, try to eat these guys raw—allinase can be deactivated by heat. Slice raw red or Vidalia onions for your sandwich or burger; chop green onions into your salad or garlic into your dressing.
- Pair garlic with olive oil to release even more helpful organosulfur compounds. Sauté the white part of leeks with garlic for a double dose of allium power.
- To battle garlic breath (which can last up to eighteen hours—gross), chew a sprig of parsley or mint after your meal. Be sure to brush and floss, and use a tongue scraper and/or mouthwash regularly.

▶ POWER NUTRIENT FOOD GROUP #3: BERRIES

Berries (BEST CHOICE) have high quantities of polyphenols, the same phytochemicals that give wine and chocolate a lot of their health-protecting qualities. But unlike wine and chocolate, berries are not fattening and have no caffeine. Berries owe their beautiful colors to anthocyanins, flavonoids that just might trip our fat-burning genes in the right direction. One Japanese researcher found that anthocyanins stop individual fat cells from getting larger and encourage fat cells to release adiponectin, a hormone that helps reduce inflammation, lower blood sugar, and reverse leptin and insulin resistance. Another study found that anthocyanins can reduce blood glucose levels after starch-rich meals, preventing insulin spikes that lead to diabetes. Certain polyphenols found in raspberries and strawberries block the digestive enzyme activity of specific starches and fats, reducing your body's absorption of them. Combine this activity with the soluble fiber in berries, and you have a sweet treat that works hard to help you lose weight and keep your blood sugar where you want it—low.

HORMONE TRIGGER FOODS: TESTOSTERONE

On the Master Your Metabolism diet, except in the case of PCOS, we are in the testosterone-boosting business, whether you're a girl or a guy. Testosterone gives us energy, builds muscle, makes us randy. It also helps protect our bones and our brains—all good stuff. And if we take advantage of the many ways our food can help us boost testosterone, we may never have to consider supplementing.

Testosterone Reducers	Why	Sources and Solutions
Alcohol	A study found that alcohol reduced testosterone levels in men.	Alcoholics who gave up drinking saw their testosterone levels go up after 6 weeks of sobriety. One more reason to hold yourself to a drink a day.
Licorice	Licorice blocks enzymes responsible for creating testosterone (although some studies have shown that the decrease is not very significant).	The occasional piece of black licorice is not going to kill your sex drive, but don't make it a regular habit.
Low-fat diet	A low-fat diet blunts the normal rise in testosterone after lifting weights. (Don't forget that testosterone is built from cholesterol, a form of fat.)	Make sure your postworkout snack contains a good balance of fat and protein.
Low-protein diet	A study of older men found that a low-protein diet elevated sex hormone–binding globulin (SHBG) levels. Since SHBG binds to other hormones and makes them unavailable for use, elevated SHBG decreases available testosterone.	Stick with the 30 percent protein ratio in this diet. (See chapter 7.)
Phytoestrogens, specifically lignans	Declines are very small, but a study found that eating foods with phytoestrogens lowers testosterone. One study found that in women, lignans lower testosterone.	Flaxseed oil is high in lignans—try to get most of your omega-3s from fish oil rather than this vegetarian source.

Testosterone Raisers	Why	Sources and Solutions
Allicin	A study on rats found that garlic coupled with a high-protein diet increased testosterone levels. Allicin also inhibits cortisol, which can compete with testosterone and interfere with its normal function.	Add some garlic and sliced onions to your burgers to boost testosterone's effect.
B vitamins	B vitamin intake was shown to correlate with elevated levels of testosterone.	You can get plenty of Bs in fortified cereals, beans, meat, poultry, and fish.
Caffeine	A study found that high doses of caffeine coupled with exercise can boost testosterone levels.	Tempting though it may be to use this as an excuse for your daily joe fix, data regarding the effect of regular intake of caffeine on testosterone is lacking. Stick with 1 to 2 caffeinated beverages a day, and finish them before noon.
Niacin	Niacin has been shown to boost HDL. High HDL levels are associated with higher testosterone levels.	Niacin is found in many foods, including dairy products, lean meats, poultry, fish, nuts, and eggs. In addition, many breads and cereals have niacin added to them.
Vegetable fat	Vegetable fat intake was shown to increase dihydrotestosterone, a form of testosterone responsible for body hair growth.	Take it easy on the soybean, corn, safflower, and sunflower oils; get your vegetable fats from canola and olive oil instead.
Zinc	One study found that restricting zinc in healthy young men led to a 75 percent reduction in their testosterone, but supplementing zinc-deficient older guys doubled their testosterone.	You can find zinc in lots of great protein foods, such as oysters, Dungeness crabs, beef, pork, dark meat chicken and turkey, yogurt, Cheddar cheese, cashews, almonds, baked beans, and garbanzos.

Hormone Homework: *Have at least 1 serving per day (as much as you can afford!)*

- Organic is a must! Berries are among the most pesticide-laden fruits.
- Fresh or frozen is best. You lose almost all the anthocyanins when you eat berries in processed foods.
- Look for packages with no visible juice stains, which suggest the berries are past their prime. Discard any soft or bruised berries and store the rest in a bowl lined with a paper towel in the refrigerator. Try to eat them within forty-eight hours of purchase.
- When berries are in season at the local farmers market, buy an entire flat, take them home, and gently wash them and let them dry. Place the berries on a cookie sheet and freeze them, then transfer them to a freezer-safe bag, where they can keep for up to two years.
- Black raspberries have an extremely high concentration of anthocyanins and ellagic acid and can often be found growing wild—keep your eyes peeled!

POWER NUTRIENT FOOD GROUP #4: MEAT AND EGGS

Did you cringe a little when I said you'd be eating foods that grew from the ground or had a mother? This is the mother part. On this plan, you're going to eat meat. All different kinds, but primarily those high in beneficial fats, like CLAs or omega-3s.

Meat is the best source of the amino acids you need to build muscle (BEST CHOICE: Alaskan wild salmon). Meat and eggs both have amino acid L-arginine, critical to the production of protein and to the release of growth hormone in the body. L-arginine is also a precursor to nitric oxide (NO), a beneficial gas that improves the functioning of your endothelium, the lining of your blood vessel walls, to decrease clotting and increase blood flow. (NO is the driving force behind Viagra, if you catch my meaning.)

The amino acid tyrosine not only keeps a lid on your appetite and reduces body fat, it also supports the healthy function of your thyroid, pituitary, and adrenal glands. Leucine, another amino acid found in meat, eggs, and fish, also helps the body produce growth hormone, as well as regulate blood sugar levels and grow the muscles that help all your hormones work better, especially insulin and testosterone.

You know those twenty-five years of trying to reduce dietary cholesterol to keep blood cholesterol levels down? Yeah, forget that. All sex steroids are created from cholesterol, so your body needs the cholesterol in meat and eggs to make that precious testosterone. In fact, many experts now believe there is little connection between dietary cholesterol and unhealthy blood cholesterol. (Oops, their bad.) Turns out whole eggs are a nearly perfect food, with almost every essential vitamin and mineral our bodies need to function. (Pair an egg with an orange and you'll get the one thing that's missing—vitamin C.)

Protein increases your metabolic rate because it takes more energy to burn than carbs or fats. When you eat protein and fat, especially the omega-3s found in organic free-range eggs, meat, and fatty deep-sea fish, ghrelin levels drop and the stomach releases more of the neuropeptide CCK, slowing down digestion and lowering your appetite. Salmon, which is rich in omega-3s, is also a source of selenium, which is critical to your thyroid, and vitamin D, which helps to preserve muscle.

Salmon is also the perfect food when you have PMS: One serving of salmon gives you a huge amount of tryptophan, the precursor to serotonin, a brain chemical associated with calm and positive moods. And eating fish also helps to reduce your body's production of prostaglandins. Prostaglandins act like hormones in the body, but rather than move their messages around the bloodstream, they stay right in the cells. You can blame prostaglandins for inflammation, pain, and fever in your body— and cramps. But while omega-6 fatty acids produce prostaglandins, salmon's omega-3 fatty acids can help blunt their effects.

The omega-3s in salmon and organic free-range meats and eggs also help to manage blood sugar and fight obesity. A dose of 1.8 grams of eicosapentaenoic acid (EPA) a day—most easily achievable with fish oil capsules—has been shown to increase adiponectin levels, increasing insulin sensitivity. Another study suggests that fish may help the body become more sensitive to leptin and less likely to become leptin-resistant.

Many vegetarians might argue that you can get omega-3s from vegetable sources, but no plant source of omega-3s would ever get you close to this beneficial dose. Our bodies convert only 5 percent of ALA omega-3s (from flaxseed, walnuts, and other tree nuts) to EPA, and even less to DHA. By all means, include these in your diet, but don't count on them to get you to a desirable threshold for healthy fats. For that, don't mess around—eat organic meat, eggs, fatty fish, and, for good measure, take mercury-free fish oil capsules. Because we have to face the one huge, unavoidable bummer of fish: toxins. Were it not for that, you could eat fish every day of the week and I'd be happy—and so would your hormones.

If you live in the modern world, you have no need to try to boost your cortisol—that's probably done for you on a daily basis. Your focus instead will be on trying to keep levels of this fat-storing hormone low. For some of us, fighting stress with food is a natural state of affairs. But we're not talking Dove bars and potato chips here—many healthy foods help you lower cortisol, so that you can lose weight rather than gain it.

Cortisol Reducers	Why	Sources and Solutions
High-fiber foods	Carbohydrates, but more specifically, dietary fiber, lowers cortisol. High-fiber carbs don't cause an insulin spike so epinephrine levels don't spike either.	Foods high in soluble fiber include oat bran, oatmeal, beans, peas, rice bran, barley, citrus fruits, strawberries, and apple pulp. Foods high in insoluble fiber include whole wheat breads, wheat cereals, wheat bran, cabbage, beets, carrots, Brussels sprouts, turnips, cauliflower, and apple skin.
Phosphatidylserine (BSE)	A natural chemical that buffers overproduction of cortisol in response to physical stress	Mackerel, herring, eel, tuna, chicken, beans, beef, pork, whole grains, green leafy vegetables, and rice
Plant sterols	A double-blind study showed that when plant sterols were given to marathon runners before a race, their cortisol levels did not rise (unlike the placebo group, which did have elevated levels), indicating reduction in the adrenal stress response.	You can get plant sterols in fortified table spreads and salad dressings, such as the Smart Balance brand, but they're by no means mandatory on this diet—after all, they are processed foods.
Vitamin C	Studies done on animals found that vitamin C prevented a rise in cortisol and protected them from other physical signs of stress. Cortisol levels were three times as high in animals that did not receive vitamin C. Since vitamin C is released from the adrenals during stress, extra vitamin C could help support this important gland.	All fruits and vegetables contain some amount of vitamin C. The highest sources include green peppers, citrus fruits and juices, strawberries, tomatoes, broccoli, turnips and other leafy greens, sweet potatoes, and cantaloupe.
Whey protein	The tryptophan in whey protein increases serotonin, lowering cortisol and enhancing your ability to deal with stress.	Try adding whey protein powder to shakes.

Cortisol Raisers	Why	Sources
Alcohol	Alcohol activates the hypothalamic-pituitary-adrenal (HPA) axis, causing the adrenals to produce more cortisol.	Studies show that heavy drinking brings up cortisol levels. One study did find that a glass of white wine actually lowers cortisol. Bottom line: Stick to one or less drink a day.
Caffeine	Caffeine increases cortisol secretion by elevating production of adrenocortico-trophic hormone (cortisol's precursor) at the pituitary.	The key here is moderation. No more then 200 milligrams a day total.
Capsaicin	Capsaicin causes the adrenal glands to secrete epinephrine, norepinephrine, and cortisol, but only for about 15 minutes. An hour after this brief rise your adrenal hormones may sink lower than they began, possibly because of an endorphin release.	Many studies have linked capsaicin-rich cayenne to lowered pain, inflammation, and risks of heart disease, cancer, and stomach ulcers, so this cortisol raiser is one to keep.
Gluten	Gluten intolerance leads to elevated cortisol levels. Many people are gluten-intolerant and don't know it.	If you're concerned, look for gluten-free products; more companies are listing them on their labels every day. Or just try to reduce the amount of wheat products you consume.
Licorice	Glycyrrhetinic acid in licorice inhibits an enzyme that inactivates cortisol in the kidneys. Eating licorice essentially extends the lifetime of cortisol in the kidneys.	Steer clear of licorice, and definitely skip the red Twizzlers, made almost entirely out of corn.
Salt	Sodium intake modifies an enzyme that helps turn cortisone into cortisol.	Since 77 percent of our sodium comes from eating prepared or processed foods, your switch to fresh foods will help you stay within a range of 1,500 to 2,400 mg of sodium a day.

Go figure: Those codes on your fruits' labels actually mean something. You'll not only learn where the fruit was grown, you'll also learn *how* it was grown. Here's a handy chart to help you decipher them, so that you can avoid any endocrine-disrupting junk.

Number on Label	What It Means	Example
Four numbers	The fruit was conventionally grown.	4011—conventionally grown yellow banana
Five numbers, beginning with 9	The fruit was organically grown.	94011—organic banana
Five numbers, beginning with 8	The fruit was genetically engineered.	84011—genetically engineered banana

Hormone Homework: *Have 3 to 5 servings (from recommended sources) per week.*

- Always buy wild-caught salmon—farm-raised salmon are fed a diet that raises their omega-6s, not their omega-3s. Farmed fish have higher levels of PCBs and other organochlorines than wild-caught, and their farms create sea lice that kill wild salmon. (Go to www.mbayaq.org for the best choices in seafood for your area.)
- Eat fish within two days of purchase. If you can't find wild salmon in your area, consider ordering it online—it's worth the investment and the peace of mind.
- Used canned salmon, which is almost always wild-caught, to sprinkle over salads, fold into a wrap, or add to an omelet. Or try kippered snacks—smoked herring, quite delicious all by itself—or sardines.
- Pasture-raised, grass-fed beef has a stronger flavor than corn-fed—some love it, but it can take some getting used to.
- If you're really freaked out about the environmental toxins in fish, you can (and should!) take a daily fish oil supplement instead.

> ## POWER NUTRIENT FOOD GROUP #5:
> ## COLORFUL FRUITS AND VEGETABLES

By seeking out vegetables of varying colors (BEST CHOICE: tomatoes), you'll automatically get a range of phytonutrients, each of which has its own particular health-promoting strengths. These colorful plant foods also happen to be incredible sources of soluble and insoluble fiber—both essential for hormone balance and impossible to get from animal products.

When people think "vegetables," they often think of greens. Some of the most powerful leafy and cruciferous veggies are green, and we'll address them below. But some of my favorites are the vibrant-colored vegetables in orange, yellow, red, and purple. The UCLA Center for Human Nutrition's color-code system divides vegetables into several distinct color groups; I've adapted their system here.

Orange: Foods high in beta-carotene include many orange vegetables, such as carrots, sweet potatoes, cantaloupe, and mangoes. Researchers believe beta-carotene may help cells speak with one another a bit more fluently, increasing the body's ability to avoid cancer. Beta-carotene also plays an important role in the production of progesterone during pregnancy.

Yellow: Most citrus foods fall into this category, and the vitamin C in citrus can also help us to manage stress. One German study made subjects stand in front of a huge group of people and do math problems. Those who had received 1 gram of vitamin C had much less cortisol and lower blood pressure than those who had not.

Purple: We talked about some of the powerhouse purples in the berry section. Other purple fruits and vegetables, including grapes and olives, have high levels of resveratrol, a type of plant antibiotic with tremendous promise in antiaging, anti-inflammatory, and blood-sugar-lowering effects. Even when rats were fed diets high in hydrogenated trans fats, resveratrol reduced their risk of death by 30 percent.

Red: All red fruits and veggies share the phytochemical lycopene, a powerful cancer-fighting antioxidant. Several studies found that those men with the highest blood levels of lycopene had the lowest risk of developing prostate cancer. Lycopene also halts oxidative stress, the process by which LDL particles harden and gunk up the arteries. When healthy adults avoided lycopene for two weeks, their fat oxidation jumped by 25 percent. One of the richest sources of lycopene on the colorful vegetable and fruit list actually qualifies as *both:* the tomato. One cup of tomatoes gets you almost 60 percent of your daily value of vitamin C for just thirty-seven calories. You might not imagine it, but tomatoes are also a very good source of fiber: one cup yields almost 8 percent of your daily needs and helps you counter high blood sugar.

Hormone Homework: *Have 5 servings per day.*
- Try for at least one serving from each color category each day to get a good balance of varied phytonutrients.
- Fruit salads, salsa, smoothies, tossed salads—any dishes that include a rainbow of color help you in your colorful fruit and vegetable allotment for the day.
- Cooking tomatoes concentrates their power: tomatoes heated for two minutes in-

Many fish are excellent sources of omega-3s, but you do have to watch out for heavy metals and other toxicity. Fish caught in rivers near Pittsburgh had so much exogenous estrogen floating in their bodies that extracts of their cells caused cancer cells to grow in the lab. One gram of fish fat also contains an average of five to twenty times as much PCBs and dioxin as an equal amount of other animal fat. PCBs have been traced to lower IQ scores, poor memory and attention, and thyroid dysfunction.

Stay safe. The folks at Seafood Watch at the Monterey Bay Aquarium have created great regional seafood guides (www.mbayaq.org)—check out the best choices, for both environmental and health reasons, for your area. Here are my suggestions for the best and worst choices for fish:

Go with These	Stay Away from These
Abalone	Atlantic cod
Alaska wild salmon (fresh, frozen, or canned)	Atlantic flounder/sole
Anchovies	Blue and king crab
Atlantic char	Bluefin tuna
Atlantic herring	Bluefish
Atlantic mackerel	Chilean sea bass
Barramundi (U.S.-farmed, not imported)	Croaker
Black sea bass	Eel
Clams (steamers)	Grouper
Halibut	King mackerel
Oysters (farmed)	Lingcod
Pacific cod	Marlin
Pacific halibut	Orange roughy
Pacific pollock	Pacific roughy
Pacific rockfish	Shad
Rainbow trout (farmed)	Shark
Sablefish	Summer and winter flounder
Sardines	Swordfish
Snapper	Wahoo
Stone, Kona, and Dungeness crab	White sea bass
Tilefish	Wild striped bass
Tuna (canned light or albacore from the United States and Canada)	Wild sturgeon

creased their lycopene and antioxidant activity by 50 percent; thirty minutes increased them by 150 percent. Choose organic sauce, paste, ketchup—all have greater lycopene content with no HFCS.

- In contrast, many other colorful veggies lose their potency with cooking. Eat a combination of raw and cooked vegetables to cover all bases.
- When in doubt, keep the skin on. Lots of insoluble fiber hides in that carrot, apple, or pear skin.
- Shop for produce in season, and always look for organic first. Check out www.local harvest.org for a market near you or sign up for a subscription to a CSA (community-sponsored agriculture) farm (www.localharvest.org/csa). If you're concerned about your food bill, check the list of essential organic choices on page 151.
- Fall in love with low-sodium tomato juice, very low in calories but incredibly filling—one six-ounce serving gives you 33 milligrams of vitamin C for only thirty calories.
- If you're in a rush, buy some fresh salsa—*without* preservatives—from the produce section of the grocery store. Eat a cup with lunch and get tomatoes, peppers, and onions all at the same time.

POWER NUTRIENT FOOD GROUP #6: CRUCIFEROUS VEGETABLES

When you chew cruciferous vegetables (BEST CHOICE: broccoli), you release enzymes that start the chemical process that gives these vegetables their unbeatable cancer-fighting properties. The byproducts of this process, isothiocyanates, are like little assassins in the body, eliminating carcinogens before they can cause genetic damage and helping to prevent bladder, cervical, colon, endometrium, lung, and prostate cancer. They can even correct problems in hormone metabolism, such as preventing estrogen from stimulating breast cancer cells.

Add to this that sulforaphane, found in cruciferous vegetables such as broccoli, cabbage, and cauliflower, was shown to help your body repair itself from damage brought on by diabetes. Sulforaphane can help your blood vessels defend against damage caused by hypoglycemia. Researchers believe these compounds can also help prevent the heart disease that often comes with diabetes.

Don't forget our nutrient density credo—these babies pack this serious nutritional power in spite of having fewer calories in every mouthful, primarily because of their high water and fiber content. That fiber fills you up and can increase your body's ability to burn fat by up to 30 percent.

Studies have consistently shown that people who eat the most fiber gain the least amount of weight.

HORMONE TRIGGER FOODS: LEPTIN

Leptin is released from your fat cells after you eat to tell your body to stop feeling hungry and start burning calories. So more should be good, right? But the fatter your body, the more leptin you produce, and your body starts to become resistant.

The goal is to optimize your leptin levels by choosing foods that work to increase your body's sensitivity to leptin, strategically raise it when necessary, and choose foods that work with other hormones to normalize your leptin functioning. Take a look.

Leptin Raisers	Why	Sources and Solutions
All omega-3s	Consistently high levels of leptin can get your metabolism in a rut, but eating omega-3 fatty acids may cause a brief dip in leptin levels and thus kick-start your metabolism.	Fatty fish like salmon, walnuts, olive oil, eggs fortified with omega-3s, and flaxseed
Eicosapentaenoic acid, or EPA (a type of omega-3)	EPA, like insulin, stimulates leptin production by increasing the metabolism of glucose.	Found in cold-water fish, such as wild salmon (*not* farm-raised), mackerel, sardines, and herring
Protein	A study found that increasing protein improved leptin sensitivity, which resulted in overall lowered calorie intake.	Up your protein to 30 percent of your daily calories. Good sources include yogurt, Pacific wild salmon, turkey, eggs, and peanut butter.
Zinc	Similar to EPA, zinc can raise leptin levels.	Oysters contain more zinc per serving than any other food, but red meat and poultry provide the majority of zinc in the average diet. Other good sources include beans, nuts, certain seafood, whole grains, fortified breakfast cereals, and dairy products.

Leptin Reducers	Why	Sources and Solutions
A huge dinner	A study found that eating an entire day's calories at dinner delayed leptin release until 2 hours after the meal.	Never eat all your calories at dinner—spread them throughout the day in 3 meals and 1 snack to help optimize leptin levels.
Alcohol	The body might sweep up leptin with the alcohol and dispose them both in the liver or kidneys.	Hold yourself to 1 glass of heart-healthy red wine a day, if desired.
Caffeine	A study found that high-caffeine consumers had low leptin levels. Once they lost weight, their leptin levels went up, but they still regained more weight than those who started with less caffeine.	If you're trying to keep weight off, avoid drinking 3 to 4 cups of coffee per day, as was consumed in the study—stick with 1 to 2 caffeine servings per day.
Fructose	Insulin tells the body to produce leptin, but unlike other sugars, fructose doesn't stimulate insulin, and thus the body doesn't release leptin. Recent animal research suggests that high fructose consumption causes leptin resistance.	Soda and candy, of course, but check food labels for the worst fructose offender: high-fructose corn syrup (HFCS), linked in animal studies to diabetes and high cholesterol
High-fat, triglyceride-raising food	Inhibits transport of leptin across the blood-brain barrier	Reduce the saturated fat, trans fat, cholesterol, and simple carb content of your diet.

Hormone Homework: *Have 2 to 3 servings per day.*
- Don't cook broccoli on the stove—microwave it instead. You'll preserve 90 percent of the vitamin C, versus 66 percent with boiling or steaming.
- Try not to overcook cruciferous veggies—not only will they be less nutritious, they can get stinky (it's the sulfur), mushy, and yucky. Try blanching them instead—throw them into a pot of boiling water for two minutes, drain quickly, and rinse with ice-cold water.
- When you bring cruciferous veggies home from the farmers market, wash and cut them right away, put them in bowls of water, and store in the fridge for instant snacks.
- Grab bags of precut broccoli, cauliflower, and cabbage at the store. Throw them into salads, eat them with hummus, fold them into burritos.

WHAT'S THE DIFFERENCE BETWEEN SOLUBLE AND INSOLUBLE FIBER?

Insoluble fiber gives our stools bulk and helps maintain regular digestion. Important benefits, sure, but soluble fiber may be more critical for hormone balance. Soluble fiber traps carbohydrates to slow their digestion, blunts the rise of glucose after meals, and keeps insulin levels low. Soluble fiber's sticky quality also helps to drag cholesterol out of the digestive tract, lowering your LDL. Experts at the University of Michigan Cancer Center say the best way to tell the difference between soluble and insoluble fiber is to picture the food submerged in water. Insoluble fiber, like an apple skin or a stalk of celery, will retain its shape; soluble fiber, found in foods like oatmeal and the inside of beans, will get gooey and sludgy. (Bonus: Most sources of soluble fiber have insoluble fiber, too.)

SOURCES OF SOLUBLE FIBER

Almonds	Cantaloupe	Pears
Apples	Carrots	Peas
Apricots	Crushed psyllium seeds	Plums
Artichokes	(Metamucil)	Potatoes
Avocadoes	Figs	Prunes
Bananas	Grapefruit	Raspberries
Barley	Ground flaxseed	Rice bran
Beans (black, garbanzo,	Kiwi	Rye
kidney, navy, pinto)	Lentils	Strawberries
Blackberries	Mangoes	Sunflower seeds
Black raspberries	Nectarines	Sweet potatoes
Broccoli	Oat bran	Tomatoes
Brussels sprouts	Oatmeal	Wheat germ
Bulgur	Onions	
Cabbage	Oranges	

- Even if you're just opening the occasional can of (healthy!) soup for dinner, toss in some chopped cruciferous veggies: cabbage, kale, rutabaga. You won't even taste them, but you'll have more volume to eat for practically zero calories, and your body will get the good phytochemicals.
- Roasted cauliflower is awesome! Place florets on a baking sheet with a light drizzle of olive oil, salt, and pepper. Bake for forty-five minutes at 450 degrees. Shake once or twice while cooking to even out the browning. Yum.

POWER NUTRIENT FOOD GROUP #7: DARK-GREEN LEAFY VEGETABLES

More than one thousand plants have leaves we can eat—but how many *do* we eat? If we eat just five servings a day, we cut our risk of developing diabetes by 20 percent. Several studies have found that leafy greens (BEST

CHOICE: spinach), more so than other vegetables, play a significant role in decreasing our risk of diabetes, possibly because of their fiber and magnesium, which helps thyroid hormone secretion, metabolism, and overall nerve and muscle function. The manganese in green leaves is also essential for normal glucose metabolism.

The vitamin C in leafy greens can be helpful to the adrenal glands as well. The adrenals release vitamin C during stress, but taking megadoses of it may lead to an increased risk of diabetes. The best way to get your vitamin C is through natural sources, such as romaine lettuce and turnip greens, both excellent choices.

If your thyroid is at all compromised, take it easy with cruciferous veggies. Perhaps because of the goitrogenic nature of isothiocyanates, very high consumption of cruciferous veggies has been linked in animal studies to an increased risk of hypothyroidism. The chances of this happening to someone without a thyroid issue is pretty slight, but if you are thyroid-sensitive, cook your cruciferous vegetables and sprinkle them with iodized salt, to counter the ions that might compete with the iodine for space in your thyroid.

The high levels of iron in spinach and Swiss chard are great for bringing oxygen to your muscles. When you don't have enough, your metabolism takes a big hit. By blocking the formation of prostaglandins, leafy greens also help prevent system-wide inflammation, reducing arthritis pain and blood clotting. The soluble fiber in dark-green leafy veggies is considered a "prebiotic," which means it helps to feed the "good" probiotic bacteria in your gut, also known to prevent inflammation.

Believe it or not, leafy greens even contain a very small amount of omega-3 fats. On their own, they won't get you all the omega-3s you need, but one serving of spinach will give you half the amount in a serving of canned tuna, and even a gram of protein.

Hormone Homework: *Have 3 to 4 servings per day.*
- Start with *arugula* and make your way through the alphabet to *turnip greens*—you'll be surprised at how delicious and different-tasting they all are.
- Start every dinner with a salad. Shake it up—do leaf lettuce one week, romaine the next. Starting this way takes the edge off your hunger, and makes sure you fit in your leafy greens. A salad plate easily holds two cups—and you're halfway to your daily goal. Add other vegetables or just a simple balsamic vinaigrette to the leaves themselves and you're golden.
- Buy frozen spinach (organic, if possible) in those little bricks—they're perfectly portioned for a full family or for an evening's meal with leftovers the next day. Sauté with olive oil, chopped garlic, and lemon.

- Use baby spinach for salads and mature spinach for cooking.
- Mesclun is actually a mix of greens including different lettuces, radicchio, dande-lion greens, endive, and others. Try mixes from different stores—all have different varieties of greens. Wash it, pat it dry with a paper towel, and use within five days of purchase.

▶ POWER NUTRIENT FOOD GROUP #8: NUTS AND SEEDS

When my clients are weaning themselves off yucky trans fat snacks, I turn them on to raw nuts like almonds, pecans, or walnuts. Nuts and seeds hit all the right snacking notes (BEST CHOICES: almonds and walnuts), yet behind the scenes, they're helping to protect you from heart disease, diabetes, and inflammation.

The Adventist Health Study found that eating nuts on a regular basis cuts your overall risk of heart attack by 60 percent. Much long-term re-search has credited omega-3s, antioxidants, fiber, L-arginine, and magne-sium with a role in helping to tamp down inflammation—and all of these precious nutrients can be found in nuts. When people eat nuts, they tend to have lower levels of C-reactive protein (CRP) and interleukin-6 (IL-6), both markers of inflammation.

Many people are afraid of nuts because of their fat; I'm more con-cerned about their calories. Perhaps both fears are groundless: Research suggests that people who eat nuts twice a week are much less likely to gain weight than those who don't eat nuts. Pine nuts are especially good at helping to prevent hunger because they stimulate the gut to produce the satiety hormone CCK.

Seeds also help reduce the risk of diabetes, as they are a source of re-sistant starch, just like beans. Resistant starch helps reduce blood sugar and dampen insulin spikes after eating. Flaxseed, in particular, is a great source of the vegetable-based omega-3, alpha-linolenic acid (ALA), which also prevents inflammation. Pumpkin seeds are a good source of omega-3s as well as zinc, a key component in testosterone production and prostate health.

Hormone Homework: *Have 1 to 2 servings per day.*
- Crush flaxseeds before you eat them; otherwise they'll pass through your digestive sys-tem without being absorbed. Store crushed seeds in the fridge to avoid oxidation.

- Try to eat raw nuts whenever possible—roasting the nuts can cause their precious fats to be damaged. Once you get used to them, you'll likely find them more satisfying and rich than roasted ones.

HEADS UP: High amounts of flaxseed and flaxseed oil can reduce blood clotting and promote bleeding, and may interact with drugs that that have a similar effect, such as aspirin.

- Sprinkle slivered almonds on your yogurt for a satisfying texture.
- Keep a handle on portion sizes—nuts are healthy, but they're very high in calories. (See "How Many Nuts or Seeds in a Serving?" on page 144.)
- Get an old-school nutcracker and grab a bag of mixed nuts still in their shells. The activity of cracking the nuts is entertaining and the effort involved will slow down your eating and cut down on mindless handfuls of nuts finding their way into your mouth.

▶ POWER NUTRIENT FOOD GROUP #9: ORGANIC DAIRY

Research is piling up that shows what a critical role dairy's calcium plays in weight control (BEST CHOICE: organic low-fat plain yogurt). Even small deficiencies of calcium change fat-burning signals in the cells and have a dampening effect on metabolism. But calcium doesn't just impact weight—a study of nine thousand people in the journal *Circulation* suggests that calcium also protects against the development of metabolic syndrome.

Grass-fed dairy products have saturated and trans fats, but they also include the best kind: conjugated linoleic acids, or CLAs. Shown to improve body composition, CLAs help to drive fat out of fatty tissues, where it can be burned up more easily. The combination of these healthy fats with dairy's high protein also stimulates the appetite-suppressing hormone CCK. Organic free-range dairy tastes better, and has no antibiotics or hormones and more omega-3s. Bonus: The zinc in dairy also helps to support healthy levels of appetite-suppressing leptin.

Most dairy foods in this country are fortified with vitamin D, which helps the body absorb calcium. Adequate vitamin D not only helps prevent osteoporosis, it has also been linked with lower risks of cancer, type 1 and type 2 diabetes, high blood pressure, glucose intolerance, and even MS. Recent research proves that our country is incredibly vitamin D–deficient. Dairy is critical, especially if you live at a higher latitude and don't get much sun during the fall, winter, and spring.

Numerous studies have found that DHEA helps the body stay young, lean, and healthy. Because DHEA is the precursor to the steroid hormones testosterone and estrogen, keeping your levels high helps you on several fronts.

DHEA Raisers	Why	Sources and Solutions
Chromium	Chromium picolinate may increase blood DHEA levels.	Good sources of chromium include carrots, potatoes, broccoli, whole grain products, and molasses.
Dietary fat	A study on menopausal women found that the more calories from fat in a diet, the higher their DHEA levels.	Make sure to eat plenty of omega-3s from fish and CLAs from organic meat and dairy.
Glucose	Stimulates secretion of pituitary ACTH, which, in turn, stimulates adrenal steroids such as DHEA	All carbs have glucose, either alone (starch or glycogen) or paired with others (such as sucrose and lactose). Stick to whole grains, low-sugar fruits like blueberries, and other carbs that don't cause spikes in insulin levels.
Magnesium	Magnesium and DHEA levels are related, although the exact mechanism is not known.	Green vegetables such as spinach are good sources of magnesium. Some legumes (beans and peas), nuts and seeds, and whole, unrefined grains are also good sources of magnesium.
Selenium	An animal study found that adrenal DHEA levels were significantly decreased by a selenium deficiency.	Good sources include Brazil nuts, salmon, whole wheat bread, crab meat, and pork.
Vitamin E	DHEA prevents breakdown of vitamin E in the body, but an animal study found that taking vitamin E can raise its level.	Vegetable oils, nuts, green leafy vegetables, and fortified cereals are good food sources of vitamin E.

The best dairy food is, by far, yogurt, primarily because of its probiotics. Remember that you are one-tenth human, nine-tenths bug. Your gut is where most of those good bugs live—ideally *trillions* of them. The probiotics in plain organic yogurt join up with the bifidobacteria, the "good" bugs already in your gut, to help fight against infections and pro-

DHEA Reducers	Why	Sources and Solutions
Low-fat, high-fiber diet	This kind of diet lowered DHEA levels in men—but when they went back to a high-fat diet, DHEA levels went back up. This effect is possibly because fiber may reduce reabsorption of DHEA once it has been excreted through the liver.	Rather than try to lower your fiber intake, which is so critical to health, instead focus on increasing your healthy fat intake from omega-3s and CLAs.
Soy isoflavones	When men with prostate cancer were given soy isoflavones, their DHEA levels dropped 32 percent.	Don't eat products with concentrated isoflavones. Choose small quantities of fermented soy, like tofu, tempeh, and miso.

tect you from yeast overgrowth. Bifidobacteria also digest the foods we eat, creating critical vitamins, including enzymes that metabolize cholesterol and bile acid. Without these microbes, the whole digestive system would squeak to a halt.

Hormone Homework: *Have 1 to 2 servings per day.*
- Take your milk straight—one 8-ounce glass of organic low-fat milk has 290 milligrams of calcium—almost a third of your daily needs—and more than 8 grams of protein.
- Don't drink chocolate or other flavored milks. And steer clear of soy milk—while it's high in calcium, it's also high in potentially dangerous phytoestrogens.
- Look for brands of yogurt (and occasionally ice cream) with no artificial preservatives, colors, flavorings, sugar, and other sweeteners—organic is best.
- Wean yourself from sugared (or, god forbid, artificially sweetened) yogurts by adding ¼ cup of plain, then ½ cup, then ¾ cup, to your regular yogurt. Once you get to 100 percent plain, use strawberries, raspberries, and blackberries to sweeten your yogurt.
- Steer clear of low-fat dairy products with thickeners and gums—I'd rather you eat a small dollop of real sour cream or a reasonable portion of full-fat cottage cheese than confuse your hormones with synthetic gunk.
- Experiment with other kinds of cultured dairy, such as buttermilk, kefir, or crème fraîche. Each of these dairy products has the distinctive tang of fermentation—your belly bugs will love you for it.
- Try high-protein Greek-style yogurt—the thicker consistency comes from being strained through muslin so the watery part is removed.
- Go easy on the full-fat cheese—it's tasty, sure, but don't forget that that taste packs a pretty hefty caloric wallop.

HOW MANY NUTS OR SEEDS IN A SERVING?

You're pretty savvy—you must be thinking, "Wait a sec, aren't nuts superfattening?" Indeed, nuts are high in calories; however, when eaten in moderation they help to combat overeating and hunger due to their fiber and protein content. Keep an eye on your portion sizes and you'll do just fine.

Type of Nut or Seed	Serving Size
Almonds	20–24
Brazil nuts	6–8
Cashews	16–18
Flaxseeds	2 tablespoons
Hazelnuts	18–20
Macadamias	10–12
Peanuts	28
Pecans	18–20
Pine nuts	150–157
Pistachios	45–47
Pumpkin seeds	85 seeds, or ½ cup
Sesame seeds	¼ cup
Walnuts	8–11 halves

Sources: www.nuthealth.org and www.calorieking.com

▶ POWER NUTRIENT FOOD GROUP #10: WHOLE GRAINS

Grains make up 25 percent of our diet—but 95 percent of that is from refined sources. That's just criminal, because whole grains can really help improve our hormone levels—and our overall health—in countless ways (BEST CHOICE: tie between oats and barley).

Most people don't realize that many whole grains are even better sources of phytochemicals and antioxidants than some vegetables, making them even more potent in the fight against heart disease and more than a dozen different kinds of cancer. Part of the power of whole grains comes from their three kinds of carbohydrate—fiber, resistant starch R1, and oligosaccharides—that skip over the small intestine so they can be fermented in the stomach. The fermentation process of these prebiotics creates beneficial short-chain fatty acids such as butyric acid. Butyric acid fights colon cancer cells while it simultaneously feeds the healthy cells of the colon. When colon cells are strong, they can help the body detox from pharmaceuticals and other environmental chemicals, just like the liver does.

The short-chain fatty acids from whole grains may also help us eat less because they stimulate fat cells in our stomachs to release leptin, the satiety hormone. The high levels of fiber in whole grains also help us feel satisfied by filling us up, slowing blood sugar release, and steadying insulin levels. For this and other reasons, eating whole grains can even help reverse insulin resistance. Epidemiological studies link high intakes of whole grain foods with lower levels of type 2 diabetes—and you need only three servings a day to reduce your risk by 30 percent.

The trick is, you have to eat grains truly whole. Even just grinding whole grains changes their cell structure and makes them more easily digested. Set your mind to it. You'll never want to go back to those refined carbs.

Hormone Homework: *Have 3 to 4 servings per day.*
- Oatmeal is the perfect breakfast—one study found that it keeps your blood sugar stable longer than many other foods. Transition away from instant varieties toward steel-cut oats, if only on the weekend.
- Try grains like amaranth, quinoa, and spelt—experiment with recipes and experience how satisfying these ancient grains can be.
- If you're buying a processed whole grain product, look at the ingredients—the whole grain should be the first one listed.
- Make the switch from semolina pasta to 100 percent whole wheat, spelt, or quinoa pasta. Give it a few tries (come on, do it!) for your taste buds to adjust to the nuttier flavor.
- Eat a whole grain cereal for breakfast—it's a fast way to get a huge jump on your soluble and insoluble fiber tally for the day. Some brands are great, but some use HFCS or NutraSweet as a trade-off for high fiber. Don't fall for it! (See the Resources on page 243 for my favorite brands.)
- Sprinkle wheat germ or bran over the top of casseroles or other baked dishes, and on yogurt and cereal.

GO ORGANIC

What is the best way you can be sure to avoid 90 percent of all hormone-disrupting agents in our food supply? **Go organic.**

Some foods are great for your thyroid function; others, not so much. If you have any issues with your thyroid, your doctor may recommend that you stay away from goitrogens, natural foods that get in the way of your thyroid's optimal functioning. (Goitrogens get their name from the goiter, a swollen thyroid gland that's struggling to produce enough hormones.) Other foods may also compound your hypothyroid issues, such as weight gain and fatigue. While the Master Your Metabolism diet is great for most, if your thyroid is out of whack, keep an eye out for these foods.

Thyroid Supporters	Why	Sources and Solutions
Deep-sea fish	Good source of omega-3s and iodine, both essential to good thyroid function	Pacific salmon, herring, sardines, anchovies
Monounsaturated fats	The thyroid needs these fats to function well.	Olive oil, avocadoes, hazelnuts, almonds, Brazil nuts, cashews, sesame seeds, pumpkin seeds
Selenium-rich foods	Helps convert thyroxine (T) to the active form (T3)	Brazil nuts, brewer's yeast, wheat germ, whole grains
Zinc-rich foods	Helps stimulate the pituitary to release TSH	Beef, lamb, sesame seeds, pumpkin seeds, yogurt, green peas, boiled spinach

Thyroid Trashers	Why	Sources and Solutions
Caffeine	Overexcites the adrenals, which may exacerbate thyroid issues	Coffee, tea, chocolate, caffeinated sodas
Goitrogenic foods	Interrupt thyroid's uptake of iodine, the building block of thyroid hormones	Millet, peaches, peanuts, radishes, strawberries, pine nuts, bamboo shoots
Raw cruciferous vegetables (cooking lessens negative effects)	Isothiocyanates disrupt normal cellular communications in the thyroid.	Brussels sprouts, cabbage, cauliflower, mustard, rutabagas, turnips, kohlrabi, collard greens, rapeseed, kale, bok choy, horseradish
Simple carbs	Resulting blood sugar crash compounds low energy from thyroid dysfunction	White pasta, white bread, refined grains, sugar, potatoes, pastries, baked goods, corn
Soy	Isoflavones may reduce thyroid hormone output by blocking critical enzyme activity.	Edamame, tofu, tempeh, textured vegetable protein, isolated soy concentrate, "not-dogs," and other faux meat products

The term "organic" applies to a farming method that raises food without pesticides or other chemicals. The idea is that by allowing natural processes and biodiversity to enrich the soil, as opposed to relying upon synthetic chemicals or genetically modified seeds to protect the crops from pests, we'll get healthier food and—imagine that—a healthier environment.

Organics help you stay slim and prevent diabetes. More than 90 percent of endocrine-disrupting pesticides that hang around in our body tissues come from foods we consume—especially animal products.

Organics help you avoid scary hormones. The FDA currently permits six kinds of steroid hormones to be used in producing cattle and sheep. Eighty percent of U.S. feedlot cattle are fed or injected with steroid hormones. Each of these cows gains up to 3 pounds *per day.*

Organics help you avoid pesticides and other chemicals. A study at the University of Washington found that the urine of kids who ate mostly conventional (i.e., pesticide-laden) diets had *nine times* the organophosphorus pesticide concentration of kids who ate mostly organic.

Organics help you prevent antibiotic resistance. Massive use of antibiotics in the meat and dairy industries leads to widespread antibiotic resistance, exposing us to potentially fatal bacteria such as methicillin-resistant *Staphylococcus aureus,* or MRSA.

Organics make your food taste better. Organic food is and will always be fresher than nonorganic food—without pesticides and chemical preservatives, organic produce has to be eaten faster or it will rot!

Organics in season make your diet more diverse. You'll switch up your fruits and veggies repertoire—asparagus in the spring, tomatoes all summer, kale and sweet potatoes in the fall—and get more phytochemicals automatically.

Organics make your food more nutritious. Organic fruits and vegetables can't rely on pesticides—they have to fight off bugs with their own "immune systems," naturally raising their antioxidant levels.

Organics help you save the earth. Produce grown in the United States travels an average of fifteen hundred miles before it gets sold. But organic farming uses 30 percent less fossil fuels while it conserves water, reduces soil erosion, maintains soil quality, and removes carbon dioxide from the air.

One quick example: Take our Power Nutrient food tomatoes. God created tomatoes and they have all the cancer-fighting health benefits

Ghrelin is a prime hunger hormone—your body releases it in anticipation of eating, whether based on your normal meal patterns or on the smell of your neighbor's barbecue. (In case you're wondering how to pronounce *ghrelin*—I did—it's "grill-en," as in, "The meat they're grillin' is making my ghrelin shoot through the roof.")

Ghrelin Reducers	Why	Sources and Solutions
Big breakfasts	People who ate a higher-calorie breakfast produced 33 percent less ghrelin throughout the day and felt satisfied for a longer period of time.	A big breakfast, like a bowl of oatmeal, half of a sliced banana, and a small low-fat yogurt
Complex carbohydrates, fiber	Insulin and ghrelin go hand in hand. If insulin goes up, ghrelin goes down.	One study found that bread was best at keeping ghrelin levels down.
Eating on a schedule	Research has found that ghrelin levels rise and fall at your usual mealtimes; eating on a schedule prevents spikes in ghrelin.	Keep some almonds or other nuts with you, so that if you're on the run, you can eat a little something at regular mealtimes.
High-volume, low-calorie foods	Levels of ghrelin remain high until food stretches the walls of your stomach, making you feel full. High-volume, low-calorie foods reduce ghrelin levels long before you've overeaten.	All green vegetables and any foods with high water content count as high-volume, low-calorie foods. Salads or soups eaten before meals will lower your ghrelin.
Protein	While not having as profound an immediate effect as carbs, protein suppresses ghrelin.	If you're not gluten-sensitive, try adding whey protein to a low-calorie smoothie. One study found that whey brought about a prolonged suppression of ghrelin.

Ghrelin Raisers	Why	Sources and Solutions
Alcohol	A study found that alcoholics have higher levels of ghrelin.	Beer, wine, and spirits—you know the drill by now
A midnight snack	A study found that night eating raises ghrelin levels. Since lower levels of ghrelin induce sleep, the higher levels from eating will actually keep you awake.	Just one of several reasons to avoid night eating. Steer clear of snacks after 9 P.M.

Ghrelin Raisers	Why	Sources and Solutions
Extremely low-calorie foods	A study found that losing one percent of your body weight results in a 24 percent increase in ghrelin levels.	Don't be tempted to lose weight quickly using meal-replacement drinks and bars. Slashing calories too dramatically will leave you hungry all the time.
Fat	Fat works in the opposite way as the carbs mentioned above—no increase in insulin means that ghrelin goes up.	Pair your protein with complex carbs to get an immediate decrease in ghrelin while you get the longer-lasting satiety that fat brings—try string cheese with half an apple.
Fructose	Unlike glucose, fructose doesn't increase insulin, which means that ghrelin will rise after you have fructose.	Check labels to avoid high-fructose corn syrup (HFCS).
Greasy, low-protein foods	Carbs suppress ghrelin fastest and deepest; protein pushes it down slower, but longer. Fats, on the other hand, are the worst—they don't suppress ghrelin nearly as well as carbs or protein, which may be another reason why high-fat diets lead to weight gain.	Deep-fried jalapeño poppers made with cream cheese—all fat, no protein. You *know* which foods to avoid.
Walking by a bakery	Your brain releases ghrelin and alerts your belly the second you see or smell food. Your stomach starts secreting digestive juices in response to sweet foods and can actually anticipate sugar, helping your body to prepare for an insulin surge.	Any high-sugar, high-calorie food that tempts you, such as cakes, candy, fresh-baked cookies; any "trigger" food that has regularly caused you to overeat

mentioned above—the best form of medicine with no harmful side effects. Now let's take our little tomato and see what happens to it in the name of capitalism. The tomato is grown conventionally, and sprayed with up to seven kinds of pesticides. Then it is picked too early because it must make the long journey across the country—or across the world—from its original location to your supermarket. Yes, you are now polluting the environment with all the gas used to transport the tomato. But there's more. The tomato is still green because it was picked too early, so now it is sprayed with argon gas (also used to euthanize dogs) to make it turn red prematurely. WOW! We have just taken God's natural medicine and turned it into poison—for us and our environment. That is why we simply must make efforts to go organic.

The more each of us votes with our dollars for products not produced with toxins, the quicker we'll help right the wrongs and get this earth back where it belongs. As more people eat organic, organic food will become cheaper.

Yeah, I knew we'd have to talk about the money.

▶ DOING THE MATH ON ORGANICS

Okay, I'll admit it. Organics can be pricey. According to the *New York Times,* organic food can be anywhere from 20 percent to 100 percent more expensive than traditionally produced foods. But the health safety issues—not to mention the environmental impact!—are too great to put a price on. And the scary research will keep piling up. Think of it this way: Every time you spend a few extra bucks to buy organic, you're saving thousands of dollars in co-pays for chemotherapy or diabetes drugs.

Also bear in mind that as demand goes up, supply will go up, and prices will go down. Most grocery chains have their own generic organic products. For example, the affordably priced Nature's Promise line (at Giant, Stop & Shop, Tops Markets, and Martin's food markets) of natural and organic meat, dairy, eggs, and frozen and fresh produce is constantly expanding. Even Wal-Mart and Target have organic store brands now.

Please always start with local options for your food—farmers markets, local organic dairies, food co-ops. But if you must shop at low-cost or big-box retailers, go for the organic instead of the conventional option. (For more tips on how to cut down on costs of organic groceries, check the "Master Shopping List" on page 236.) The Environmental Working Group (EWG) did an analysis of the most important produce to buy organic. (Check out the full list of toxic fruits and veg at www.foodnews.org.) Below you'll find their recommendations for fruits and veggies, along with mine for other foods. I'll always say go for organic, but if your pocketbook is stretched thin, use this list as your guide.

ALWAYS BUY ORGANIC

Even after washing or other attempts to reduce pesticides, these foods will remain the most toxic. Spend your organic food budget here.

1. Meat, dairy, and eggs
2. Coffee
3. Peaches and nectarines
4. Apples
5. Bell peppers
6. Celery
7. Berries
8. Lettuce
9. Grapes
10. Foods you eat a lot

SOMETIMES BUY ORGANIC

I call this the "Hey, if you've got the cash, why not?" section. Better safe than sorry.

1. Processed foods
2. Onions
3. Avocadoes
4. Pineapple
5. Cabbage
6. Broccoli
7. Bananas
8. Asparagus
9. Corn
10. Mangoes

Cows that produce organic milk are fed organic grains and are given access to pasture, but, most important, they cannot be treated with recombinant bovine growth hormone, also known as rBGH or rBST (recombinant bovine somatotropin). And thank god for that! Traditional dairy farmers feed this horrific synthetic hormone to their cows to boost their milk production, and so far, the USDA still approves them as safe. (Unlike regulatory agencies in Canada, Japan, Australia, New Zealand, and twenty-seven countries of the European Union, where rBGH is banned.)

Studies have shown that rBGH increases the levels of insulin-like growth factor 1, or IGF-1, in the milk of these cows. Drinking *just 1 glass* of milk a day for 12 weeks can increase a human's blood levels of IGF-1 by 10 percent. At normal levels, IGF-1 does good things in the body; it's responsible for cell growth, division, and differentiation. But IGF-1 has been linked, in hundreds of studies, to increased breast, prostate, uterine, colon, lung, and other cancers in humans. (Notice how many of those cancers are in sex organs?) Emerging research even links high levels of IGF-1 to autism. Rather than destroy IGF-1, pasteurization increases its levels, and because bovine and human IGF-1 are identical, this raging abundance of hormones is eagerly absorbed into the digestive tract and the bloodstream, where it can act on various parts of the body.

Awesome.

Studies have shown that high levels of IGF-1 increases ovulation. In fact, one study found that mothers who drink milk have an 80 percent greater chance of having twins. And although a link has not yet been firmly established, many believe that rBGH is one of the reasons early puberty is on the rise.

The kicker? The USDA has consistently refused to mandate that milk producers warn consumers that their milk products include rBGH, and many state dairy boards are attempting to ban any mention of rBGH on labels at all.

Still, signs are promising—Wal-Mart, Starbucks, Safeway, Kroger, and many others are starting to use rBGH-free milk. Kraft is planning a line of rBGH-free cheese. We may just get this horrific hormone banned. But in the meantime, play it safe with organic. Organic farms are third-party certified, unlike farms that produce nonorganic hormone-free milk.

DON'T BOTHER BUYING ORGANIC

Don't be duped into wasting your organic budget on

1. Seafood
2. Water
3. Foods you don't eat that often

You've Removed the toxins. You've Restored the nutrients. But exactly when and how much and in what combinations do you eat the foods on the Master Your Metabolism plan? We'll talk about that next—learning how to Rebalance the energy into your body in ways that will improve your overall hormone levels, trigger the fat-burning ones, and turn off the fat-storage ones.

CHAPTER 7

STEP 3—REBALANCE

ADJUST THE TIMING, QUANTITY, AND COMBINATIONS OF FOODS FOR MAXIMUM METABOLIC IMPACT

Thus far in the program, we've focused on the what—what foods to Remove and what foods to Restore to optimize your hormones. In this chapter, we'll focus on the how and the when to Rebalance your hormones.

The timing, quantity, and combinations of your meals have a great impact on your hormones and metabolism. This chapter will focus on when to eat what foods—and when not to—to capitalize on hormone patterns that lead to weight loss. Rebalance features three key techniques: Eat Every 4 Hours, Eat Until You're Full—But Not Stuffed, and Combine Foods Correctly. Let's take a look at each one in turn.

▶ REBALANCE TECHNIQUE #1: EAT EVERY 4 HOURS

On the Master Your Metabolism diet, you'll eat three meals and one snack: breakfast, lunch, midafternoon snack, dinner. Every day. No excuses.

I know everyone has a different way of scheduling their meals. And I want you to go with that—you know your body better than I ever will. That said, I have three iron-clad rules about meal timing that you must adhere to, or you run the risk of blowing much of the good work you've done so far:

1. You must eat breakfast.
2. You must eat every four hours.
3. You must not eat after nine P.M.—and especially never eat carbs before bed. Period.

These three rules will help you tap in to your body's natural hormonal rhythms and instinctive calorie-burning patterns. Using these techniques in combination with the Remove and Restore aspects of the plan will guarantee weight loss.

Belly up to the breakfast table. I know how some of you feel about this one, but I'm sorry, I don't want to hear it. "Jillian, I don't have time to eat in the morning." "Jillian, anything more than coffee makes me want to puke." Get over it! Less than half of us eat breakfast every day, but studies have shown that breakfast is one of the most reliable ways to achieve a healthy weight and keep your glucose and insulin steady. *In fact, women who don't eat breakfast are four and a half times more likely to be obese than women who do.* People who never eat breakfast are also the most likely to develop type 2 diabetes.

One study, published in the journal *Pediatrics,* tracked more than two thousand adolescents for five years, from the time they were fifteen until they turned twenty. Researchers found that the more often boys and girls ate breakfast, the lower their BMI. This result was independent of all other factors—age, sex, race, socioeconomic status, smoking—even whether they were concerned about their weight (and their diet). The most striking thing about this study? The kids who ate breakfast daily actually ate *more* calories than those who ate breakfast less often—but they still weighed less.

Breaking your fast jump-starts your metabolism and prevents energy sags later in the day. If you're a guy, your testosterone levels peak at about eight A.M. and reach their lowest point during the early evening. By timing your biggest meal in the morning, you'll be able to capitalize on that surge of metabolic power. One Dutch study found that people who ate a big breakfast rich in complex carbs (such as you'd get from oatmeal, high-fiber cereal, or a veggie omelet with whole grain toast) felt satisfied and full for a longer time, in part because breakfast reduced their ghrelin levels by 33 percent.

If nothing else, promise me you will always eat *something* before you work out in the morning. During the night, about 80 percent of your glycogen stores—the digested carbs waiting to be tapped as energy—

have been used up. If you work out on an empty stomach, you'll go through the last 20 percent almost immediately and then quickly begin to gobble up your lean-muscle mass—definitely not what you're trying to do here.

Hormone Homework: *Eat as early as is feasible, no more than an hour after waking up. Grab a quick bowl of high-fiber cereal or an apple with a handful of raw almonds before your workout. The sole exception to breakfast within an hour might be those taking thyroid medication—some kinds must be taken on an empty stomach, others after breakfast. Check with your doctor about the best timing for your medication and meals.*

Eat every four hours. Let me rephrase: You *must* eat every four hours. I planned the diet this way not only because eating often makes me happy but because I know it makes my metabolism happy, too. You not only don't have to live with a rumbling stomach—you shouldn't!

When you eat meals spaced four hours apart, your body doesn't get a chance to miss food, so it doesn't develop a scarcity mentality. If you feed your body every four hours, you'll prevent the massive fat storage that comes from feast-or-famine eating. (Remember that "thrifty gene" from chapter 1? We don't want to wake him up.) The act of eating and digesting accounts for 10 percent of your body's metabolic rate. Starve yourself for any portion of the day and you cheat yourself out of a good portion of this bump. The most important part of eating regularly is that it stabilizes your blood sugar and your hormones: Your blood sugar remains steady throughout the day, and because your meals are smaller, your insulin does not spike as dramatically. The body trusts that there's more where that came from, so it happily burns your meal for energy, confident that you'll feed it more later.

Additionally, by eating every four hours you keep your hunger hormone ghrelin in check and keep your leptin levels stable. These two hormones are to blame when you skip meals, become ravenous, and are much more likely to overeat. In fact, ghrelin does its job so well that when it's surging in your bloodstream, it can actually make food taste up to 20 percent better.

On the other hand, the popular concept of six small meals throughout the day is also less than ideal. You don't need your insulin surging on a constant basis by eating nonstop. Body builders developed this style of eating to squeeze thousands upon thousands of calories into their day. (How it became a weight-loss trend is beyond me.) Many of them developed type 2 diabetes later on in life. Coincidence? I think not. Eating every four hours is a perfect formula for hormone balance—it keeps insulin stable, but doesn't spike hunger hormones, either.

Hormone Homework: *When you first start to eat every four hours, believe it or not, you might find that you're not very hungry when the four hours are up. But that's the idea—we don't want you to be famished. You want to head off extreme hunger, which is a signal that your blood sugar has dipped too low, a surefire recipe for cravings and overeating.*

Don't eat after nine P.M.—especially carbs. One of the biggest risks of skipping meals during the day is that you then overeat at night. Your body uses calories throughout the day, but any big surplus gets stored as fat. One study in the journal *Metabolism* found that people who skipped meals during the day and ate a big meal between four P.M. and eight P.M. ended up with some very ominous measurements:

- Higher fasting blood glucose in the morning
- Higher blood sugar overall
- Higher levels of ghrelin
- Impaired insulin response (an indicator of insulin resistance)

Scary, right? Yet so many people I've worked with have done this—work hard all day, ignoring their need for food because they're "too busy to eat." And then, at the end of a long day, they "reward" themselves with a nice, relaxing, diabetes-inducing meal.

Your levels of fat-storage hormone cortisol dip after breakfast and lunch, but not after dinner or evening snacks. Eating more calories during the evening will pack more fat around your belly, where you have more cortisol receptors than other places in your body. Eating the bulk of your calories after dark also sends your bad LDL up and good HDL down.

The rate at which food will leave your stomach—also known as your gastric emptying rate—slows down at night. Plus, your ability to process glucose gets weaker as the day goes on. If you eat a carb-heavy meal at eight P.M., your body reacts much differently than if you eat a carb-heavy meal at eight A.M. The old adage "Eat like a king at breakfast, a prince at lunch, a pauper at dinner" is right on the money—although I'd stick another pauper in there somewhere.

The most important thing is not to eat before bed. Muscle-glycogen stores fill during the day's meals. By the end of the day, all the spots in the glycogen stores are filled up. You're not going to be burning any extra calories, or drawing on those glycogen stores, for the better part of seven or eight hours, so any remaining calories you eat now will turn straight into fat.

This part is by far the most important: About one hour after you fall asleep—at about midnight for most people—your body releases its largest pulse of growth hormone for the day. Insulin inhibits growth hormone production, so the last thing you want to do is eat any carbs that will drive up your insulin and interfere with this precious fat-burning growth hormone supply.

Hormone Homework: *As soon as you have your evening meal, shut the kitchen down and don't head there anymore. Try to make that last meal tilt more toward proteins than carbs, to keep insulin levels down and allow for maximum growth hormone release at night.*

> ### REBALANCE TECHNIQUE #2:
> ### EAT UNTIL YOU'RE FULL—BUT NOT STUFFED

This diet is not about counting calories. When you Restore nutritious foods to your diet, nature will take care of portion control for you. While you're still in the process of adopting these practices, though, consider the merits of Rebalancing your "energy in."

Eat until you're full. You need to eat enough to fuel your metabolism. As we talked about in chapter 3, when you eat too few calories, you overtax your thyroid and train your body to do more with less. And while economizing might be a good strategy for your financial health, it sucks as a dietary strategy.

That said, eating until you're full of fast food is not allowed. When you eat healthy, fresh, whole foods until you're full, you will find that your calories are within a perfect range. Not too little and not too much. For girls this is anywhere from 1,200 to 1,800. For boys this is anywhere from 1,800 to 3,000. The difference in calorie allowances has to do with age and activity level. (See "Ballpark Your Calories" on page 160.)

Severe diets make your body start eating its own muscle. Drastically reducing your calorie levels for just four days can reduce blood levels of

JUNK FOOD WITHOUT THE JUNK

I know you're human. You're going to have sugar. You're going to have chocolate. (Some argue that chocolate is a health food.) But here's the deal: Instead of a processed, artificially flavored peanut butter cup with trans fat and high-fructose corn syrup, have a Newman's Own organic peanut butter cup. Instead of a huge bowl of sugar-free, nonfat frozen yogurt, loaded with chemicals and artificial sweeteners, have half a cup of organic full-fat ice cream. If you're going to have foods that are less healthy, eat real food and not chemicals.

leptin by almost 40 percent; do it for a month and leptin plummets 54 percent. When you cut calories to lose weight, the lower your leptin levels go, the more hungry you become—a recipe for yo-yo dieting.

Eating nutrient-dense, high-fiber/high-water-content Power Nutrient foods will also help you fill up without any fear of overeating calories. As you eat these high-volume foods, your stomach starts to stretch a bit. This "distension" triggers the release of satiety peptides. Translation: You'll feel full faster, with fewer calories, and the fiber will help you stay satisfied longer. When you give your body the foods it recognizes, it eagerly absorbs the nutrients critical to optimal hormone production and puts them to work right away.

Hormone Homework: *Check out the recommended calorie range for your size and activity level. If the range is 1,200–1,400 calories, don't go down to 800—you'll damage your metabolism and inhibit your thyroid. On the other hand, don't do what some of my clients do when they hear that eating often ups their metabolism by 10 percent—they go out and order a pizza! The problem is that 10 percent for most people is about 200 calories—not 3,000! Know your range and stick close to it.*

But not until you're stuffed. Now for the bad news: If you've been eating at least one large meal a day, you probably stretched out your stomach, making it difficult to feel full and trigger your satiety hormones. You may even have leptin resistance—your body could be releasing leptin to let you know it's full, but you ignore the hormone and continue eating.

Good news: You can return to a state of balance and get your appetite back in check, but you have to follow these rules. Eating smaller meals four times a day will help shrink it back to normal size. When it does, you'll be equally satisfied but faster, with less food.

To train yourself to eat smaller portions, use a salad plate or a small bowl instead of a bigger dinner plate. Many dieting studies have proven that this advice works, possibly because of what marketing researchers at Washington University call the "partitioning effect." When people are given a hundred dollars to spend, those who receive it in ten envelopes of ten dollars each spend fifty dollars; those who are given one envelope with one hundred dollars blow the whole thing. The same effect works with food, because when you reach one partition—finishing the food on a smaller plate, say—you have to make a conscious choice to reach for more.

Compare that scenario with the mindless shoveling of food from a bigger dinner plate. We've seen how those large meals send insulin levels soaring and overtax all the systems responsible for digestion. When you take the calories eaten during one large meal and spread them throughout the day, all your cells, organs, glands, and hormones can do their jobs so much easier.

If you have been overeating, perhaps it would help to know that cutting your daily calorie intake by just 15 percent—from 2,000 to 1,700, for example—could reduce your risk of cancer. University of Texas researchers found that mice given 15 to 30 percent fewer calories inhibited the signaling power of IGF-1, diminishing excess cell growth and the development of papillomas, precancerous lesions on the skin. Researchers believe the same mechanism may be at work in as many as 80 percent of other cancers as well.

Yes, as complex as the whole picture of hormones and weight loss is, one undeniable maxim of weight loss still applies: Calories are important. Of the five thousand people in the National Weight Control Registry who've successfully maintained weight loss of at least 30 pounds, 99 percent of them had cut calories.

Okay, I had to say it. But that's the last time we'll mention it.

Hormone Homework: *The only portion sizes that really count are animal products, processed foods, starchy vegetables, and high-sugar fruits. (See "Using Your Rule of Thumb" below.) I truly don't care how many nonstarchy vegetables you eat. I'd love it if you would eat plates and plates full of them! Start your meal with veggies and you'll give your gut-based satiety hormones more time to kick in.*

▶ REBALANCE TECHNIQUE #3: COMBINE FOODS CORRECTLY

I don't know about you, but I am sick to death of the entire no-carb, low-carb, no-fat, high-fat conversation. Balance—that's all we need. Our bodies are built for balance.

BALLPARK YOUR CALORIES

I repeat: This program is not about calorie counting, it's about health—weight loss will come automatically. But it's still helpful to know what range you should be operating within, so check out these recommendations based on guidelines from the American Diabetes Association.

If you are . . .	Shoot for this many calories each day
An average-sized woman who wants to lose weight	1,200–1,400
A petite woman at your desired body weight	1,200–1,400
An average-sized, sedentary woman at your desired body weight	1,200–1,400
A larger woman who wants to lose weight	1,400–1,600
A larger, sedentary woman at desired body weight	1,400–1,600
A moderate-to-large, somewhat active woman at your desired body weight	1,600–1,900
An older man at your desired body weight	1,600–1,900
A small-to-moderate-sized man who wants to lose weight	1,600–1,900
A teen girl	1,900–2,300
A larger, active woman at your desired body weight	1,900–2,300
A small-to-moderate-sized man at your desired body weight	1,900–2,300
A teen boy	2,300–2,800
A moderate-to-large, active man at your desired body weight	2,300–2,800

From now on, you're going to include a bit of protein, fat, and carbs in every meal and snack (except the evening snack, which will focus on protein). As we talked about during our discussion of Power Nutrient foods, each individual nutrient performs a critical service to our hormone production. Take any one nutrient away and you start to slow down your metabolism.

We need fat. They're called "essential" fatty acids for a reason. We have to get these fats from our diet to avoid malnourishment. Animal and vegetable fats provide valuable, concentrated energy. They also provide the building blocks for cell membranes and a variety of hormones and hormonelike substances.

Fats slow the absorption of nutrients so that you can go longer without feeling hungry, and they aid in sugar and insulin metabolism, which helps you lose weight. Without fat, carbohydrates would take our blood sugar (and insulin) for a nonstop roller coaster ride. They act as carriers for the important fat-soluble vitamins A, D, E, and K, and all the carotenoids. Heart-healthy omega-3s help keep our triglycerides in check and may improve insulin resistance, and some fats—like CLAs— actually help us to burn stored fat from our bodies. People who tend toward insulin resistance *need* about 30 percent fat in their diet to help them lose weight; some studies have shown that when they try to lose weight by following low-fat diets, they either fail initially or can't keep the weight off long-term. Some researchers even argue that saturated fat, long maligned as the prime factor in the development of heart disease and obesity, is actually innocent, and may be beneficial to weight loss.

Okay, got it. Fat is good. Check.

We need protein. I'm pretty sure I won't have to fight with you on this one. You need protein to maintain and build muscle. Just the act of eating protein can help your body burn up to 35 percent more calories in digestion. Protein stimulates the production of the satiety hormone CCK and dampens levels of ghrelin. When carbohydrates are eaten without protein, insulin levels go through the roof.

Critics have traditionally said that higher-protein diets are unsustainable, that people will automatically rebound to carb craving. But research has not borne this out—in fact, quite the opposite. Numerous studies on higher-protein diets have now found that people who follow them are better able to sustain their weight loss for longer periods of time. They have better body compositions; they lower their cholesterol, triglyceride, blood sugar, and insulin levels; and they increase their metabolisms more than when they began. The longer you follow a diet with 30 percent protein, the more the postmeal fat-burning effects work for you. Researchers found that someone who regularly eats a 30 percent protein lunch may burn ten more extra calories per minute than the person who routinely eats less than 20 percent protein. (This effect lasts for more than three hours after you eat—just in time for your next meal!)

Even concerns about the increased heart attack risk of higher-protein diets have begun to fall apart. One Swedish study found that 66 percent of the control subjects who ate "normal" diets suffered a stroke or heart

USING YOUR RULE OF THUMB

One survey found that only 1 percent of us can gauge serving sizes correctly. Play around with measuring cups and get a feel for portion sizes. It won't take long to learn what a cup of milk looks like or how many ounces of chicken are in a small breast.

Portion	Looks like
3 ounces of meat	A child's palm or a deck of cards
5 ounces of meat	An adult's palm or 2 decks of cards
½ cup of pasta or grain	½ of a baseball (not a softball!)
1 teaspoon butter	The tip of your finger (or one die)
1 teaspoon oil	The tip of your finger (or one die)
1 tablespoon peanut butter	½ of a Ping-Pong ball
1 medium fruit	A fist or a baseball
1 ounce of cheese	Four dice
1 tablespoon dressing	½ of your thumb
1 cup of veggies	A fist or a baseball
1 bagel	A hockey puck
1 slice of bread	A cassette tape
1 cup of cereal	A fist or a baseball
1 pancake	A compact disc

attack during the four-year study, versus only 8 percent of test subjects on the higher-protein diet.

I think I like those higher-protein odds a wee bit better.

Protein is good. Check.

We need carbs. All that being said, we humans simply cannot function without carbs. Carbs give us energy; without them, we couldn't think, walk, dance, drive, or do anything. We need them to live. One study found that women who severely restricted their carbs for three days belly-flopped into a vat of carbs by the fourth day, eating 44 percent more calories from carbohydrate foods than they had initially.

Carbs give our food texture and crunch, variety and color. They make us happy, literally, by feeding our neurotransmitters. And people who eat three servings of whole grains a day are 30 percent less likely to develop type 2 diabetes.

Carbs are also the vehicles for so many of nature's disease fighters. Phytochemicals come only from plants, people—you can't get vitamin C from a bunless burger. Without carbs, we'd be sitting ducks for cancer, heart disease, metabolic syndrome, chronic inflammation, and digestive problems.

And as much as we've abused the vegetables in this country for years and years, pouring our toxic chemicals all over them, they may yet help to save us from ourselves. Eating fiber, a carbohydrate that can come only from plant sources, is one of the few ways we can help our bodies flush out the toxins that have built up in our tissues and messed with our endocrine systems for years.

Remember, the key here is GOOD CARBS! Vegetables, fruits, whole grains. You've been paying attention, right? If so, I shouldn't have to reiterate this point, but I did . . . just in case.

So, yes, we need carbs. Carbs are good. Check.

Hormone Homework: *A 40 percent carbs, 30 percent protein, 30 percent fat balance is a safe solution. Now, you can play with this ratio a little bit. Some people will find they do better with a little more carbohydrate, and some people do better with a little less. The final precise ratio for you has to do with the rate at which your body breaks down your food into energy. Fine-tuning your macronutrients can help give you more energy and keep you feeling fuller longer. I wrote entire volumes on this point in my two previous books, so I won't go into great depth here. The bottom line: You must have fat, protein, and carbs in each meal. Period.*

Scientists are just starting to appreciate how certain hormones, pesticides, and chemicals interact with one another to produce side effects exponentially more dangerous. Well, luckily for us, high-quality nutrition can have exponential effects, too.

Nature has a powerful way to fight back, a health phenomenon also greater than the sum of its parts, called "food synergy." This new field of nutrition has sprung up to study certain foods and patterns that appear to work together to combat diseases such as cancer, heart disease, and other chronic conditions in a stronger way than individual nutrients could on their own.

But I'll let you in on a little secret—food synergy is just a fancy way of saying "Eat whole foods." Don't focus on carbs, or protein, or fat—just food. Whole foods work together to bring out each nutrient's individual strengths. By eating more whole foods, you're inviting more of these natural synergies into your body, where they can work together to optimize your hormones and detox your body.

THE DIET AT A GLANCE

As long as you focus on these three main principles—and eat food that is clean, whole, and balanced—you can't go wrong:

1. **CLEAN:** First, you look for the dish with the smallest number of adulterating additives and hormone-disrupting chemicals.

REMOVE THESE FOODS

- Hydrogenated fats
- Refined grains
- High-fructose corn syrup
- Artificial sweeteners
- Artificial coloring and preservatives
- Glutamates

REDUCE THESE FOODS

- Starchy vegetables
- Tropical, dried, and canned fruits
- Excess soy
- Excess alcohol
- Full-fat dairy and fatty meats
- Canned foods
- Caffeine

2. **WHOLE:** Then you look for foods that came from the ground or had a mother.

RESTORE THESE FOODS

- Legumes
- Alliums
- Berries
- Meat and eggs
- Colorful fruits and veggies
- Cruciferous veggies

- Dark-green leafy veggies
- Nuts and seeds
- Dairy
- Whole grains

3. **BALANCED:** Finally, you get a healthy balance of protein, fat, carbs, and calories throughout the day.

REBALANCE YOUR ENERGY

- Eat breakfast
- Eat every four hours
- Do not eat after 9 P.M.
- No carbs at night

- Eat until you're full
- But not stuffed
- Eat 40 percent carbs, 30 percent fat, 30 percent protein

The special combination of steps—to Remove the hormones, pesticides, and chemicals in conventionally raised foods; to Restore lost nutrients; and to Rebalance your energy in and out—allows you to tap in to this food synergy on a daily basis. All of the plan's facets work together to bring out these hormone-optimizing foods' most powerful healing qualities. And now you're going to learn how to fit all the pieces of the program together.

PART 3

THE MASTER TOOLS

CHAPTER 8

THE MASTER LIFESTYLE STRATEGIES

REMOVE TOXINS IN YOUR HOME,
RESTORE LOST NUTRIENTS IN YOUR DIET, AND
REBALANCE ENERGY TO ERASE CRUSHING STRESS

As we've seen, our bodies are literally under assault in the modern world. Some toxins we ingest, such as refined sugars, artificial sweeteners, additives, and prescription medicines. Some come from our environment: air and water pollution, cosmetics, petrochemical and industrial wastes, and heavy metals. Some we even inflict upon ourselves: overwork, overeating, lack of sleep.

All these chemicals and habits wreak havoc on our biochemistry and cellular health. And the more of these toxic chemicals and habits we have, the greater our "bioburden," the combined impact of all of these endocrine disruptors.

Now that we've cleaned up your diet, we have to clean up everything else. We have to Remove the remaining toxins in your home, Restore any remaining nutritional deficiencies, and Rebalance your energy to fight back against the crushing stress that can send hormones reeling. By the time you're done here, you will have erased many of the remaining hormonal threats and rebooted your metabolism entirely.

But don't look at the suggestions in this chapter as one program—that would be a tall order and a lot to handle. Treat them as small steps with a cumulative effect. The suggestions in this chapter represent a best-case scenario for reducing your bioburden; if you do half of them, you'll be in great shape.

Let's get to work.

REMOVE TOXINS FROM YOUR ENVIRONMENT

Cleaner choices not only help you lose weight and look amazing, they also sustain the earth. With each change you make to your kitchen, home, or garden, you'll have that much more impact on your own metabolism, vitality, longevity, health, and happiness.

REMOVING TOXIC PLASTICS FROM YOUR HOME

Manufacturers use plastics more than any other material; some are more likely to leach endocrine disruptors and other dangerous chemicals than others. You can tell the different plastics by the numbers printed on the bottom of the containers. Let's go over the full list, so that you know which are the least toxic and which you need to stop using *now*. (Check out a list of safe and unsafe national brands at www.checnet.org/healthe House/pdf/plasticchart.pdf.)

UNSAFE PLASTICS—DO NOT USE!

These plastics are three prime suspects in the hubbub over environmental estrogens. Avoid them at all costs.

NO! #3—Polyvinyl chloride (V or PVC)

Found in cooking-oil bottles, cling wrap, clear wrap around meat, cheese, deli meats, and other food items, plumbing pipes, toys.

Why it's bad: Hormone-disrupting phthalates and cancer-causing dioxins leach out of PVC when it comes into contact with heat, food (especially cheese and meat), water, air, or our bodies.

Choose these instead: Glad wrap; Saran premium wrap, and Saran Cling Plus wrap do not contain PVC or bisphenol A. Store your food in glass.

Buy cooking oil in glass bottles. *Never* microwave food in plastic—use parchment paper or wax paper.

NO! #6—Polystyrene (PS; extruded type is known as Styrofoam)

The extruded type is found in disposable coffee cups, takeout containers, foam egg cartons, meat trays, packing peanuts, and foam insulation. The nonextruded type is found in CD jewel cases, disposable cutlery, and transparent takeout containers.

Why it's bad: Especially when it gets hot, known endocrine disruptor polystyrene can leach chemicals into food. Materials used to create polystyrene—benzene, butadiene, and styrene—are all known or suspected carcinogens.

Choose these instead: Buy eggs packaged in cardboard containers. Transfer foods packed in polystyrene to glass or ceramic containers as quickly as possible. Never drink hot drinks out of foam cups or eat food out of foam containers. Go to restaurants that use paper-based takeout containers and corn- or sugar-based disposable cutlery and cups.

NO! #7—Other (PC, for polycarbonate)

Found in baby bottles, microwave ovenware, stain-resistant food-storage containers, medical storage containers, eating utensils, plastic liners of almost all food and soft-drink cans, Lexan containers, old Nalgene or other hard-plastic drinking bottles, five-gallon water jugs, building materials.

Why it's bad: Hundreds of studies on animals and humans have linked bisphenol A (BPA), a chemical in polycarbonate plastic, with harmful endocrine-disrupting effects, such as early puberty in girls, abnormal breast tissue and prostate growth, and lower sperm counts.

Choose these instead: Rinse your canned food thoroughly before you eat it. Use glass baby bottles, but if you continue to use polycarbonate bottles, don't stick them in the bottle warmer—warming them increases the leaching effect. Switch to stainless steel or ceramic-lined drinking bottles. Do not wash your polycarbonate drinking bottles in the dishwasher. Once it starts to get cloudy, get rid of it. If you ever smell plastics in any water or liquid, *do not drink it.*

SAFE(R) PLASTICS

These plastics have a better track record than the three above. But if you ask me, the fewer plastics in your life, the better.

OKAY: #1—Polyethylene terephthalate (PET or PETE)

Found in bottles for cough syrup, ketchup, salad dressing, soft drinks, sports drinks, and water. Also found in plastic pickle, jelly, jam, mustard, mayonnaise, and peanut butter jars.

OKAY: #2—High-density polyethylene (HDPE)

Found in toys, shampoo bottles, milk jugs, yogurt containers, margarine tubs, recyclable grocery bags, trash bags, laundry detergent bottles, composite lumber, Tyvek building material, some Tupperware products, sanitary products, original Hula-Hoops, some shrink wrap.

OKAY: #4—Low-density polyethylene (LDPE)

Found in grocery bags, bowls, lids, toys, six-pack rings, trays, power cables, liners, some cling wrap, sandwich bags, food-coloring and other squeezable bottles, bottle caps.

OKAY: #5—Polypropylene (PP)

Found in plastic utensils, cups, thermal underwear (such as Under Armour brand), clear bags, diapers, safe baby bottles, Stonyfield Farm yogurt containers, condiment bottles.

REMOVING TOXINS FROM YOUR KITCHEN

With more than one hundred thousand chemicals out there, and very few of them studied, we'll soon see much research about how damaging more of these are. In the meantime, protect yourself in the kitchen.

NO: Chlorinated white paper towels

The EPA found that dioxins, byproducts of chlorine, are three hundred thousand times more carcinogenic than DDT; they're also very estrogenic.

YES: Chlorine-free paper products

Use products—toilet paper included—that say they are processed chlorine-free, or PCF.

KEEP THE DISHWASHER CLOSED

Don't open your dishwasher door during the wash cycle. That "whoosh" of steam releases toxic volatized chlorine from the combination of detergent and tap water.

NO: Bleached coffee filters

Bleached coffee filters leach chlorine into your coffee and release dioxins with every drip.

YES: Unbleached or oxygen-bleached filters

These use chlorine dioxide, a type of bleach that doesn't create dioxin residues.

NO: "Antibacterial" dish soap (or anything!)

In addition to helping create antibiotic resistance, when triclosan combines with chlorinated tap water, it creates the carcinogenic gas chloroform and chlorinated dioxins, a highly toxic form of dioxin.

YES: Natural soaps

Choose dish soaps without chlorine or phosphates. Good brands include Seventh Generation, Ecover, and Mrs. Meyer's.

NO: Teflon pans

A chemical in Teflon likely damages the liver and thyroid and impairs the immune system.

YES: Iron, porcelain-coated, stainless steel, or glass pans

Get added iron as you avoid endocrine and immune-system damage.

REMOVE TOXINS FROM YOUR BATHROOM CABINET

Cosmetics and personal-care products are actually a huge source of chemical poisoning and endocrine disruption. But the FDA has tested only 11 percent of the 10,500 ingredients used in cosmetics. Thankfully, the Campaign for Safe Cosmetics, a consortium of sixty environmental and consumer health groups, identified some of the most harmful substances in cosmetics and personal-care products. When looking for alternatives, seek out companies that signed the Campaign for Safe Cosmetics compact, a pledge of their commitment to safer products and greater transparency about the ingredients of their products. A list of signing companies can be found at www.safecosmetics.org. The following ingredients all have suspected hormone-disrupting qualities.

NO: Mercury (often listed as thimerosal on ingredient labels)

Found in some lip liner, lip gloss, facial moisturizer, mascara, eye drops, ointment, and deodorant.

Why it's bad: Mercury sticks around in the tissues forever, messing with our neurochemistry, immune systems, and other cells. It is also a suspected endocrine disruptor and a known human reproductive and developmental toxin.

NO: Lead

Found in more than 60 percent of brand-name lipsticks, but never labeled as such.

Why it's bad: Lead causes learning and behavioral disorders and has been linked to other central nervous system damage, miscarriage, reduced fertility, hormonal changes, and menstrual irregularities.

NO: Toluene

Found in nail polish and other cuticle and nail treatments.

Why it's bad: Toluene damages the nervous, respiratory, and cardiovascular systems; it may also damage kidneys, lower sperm counts, cause birth defects, and interfere with normal menstrual cycles.

NO: Formaldehyde

Found in moisturizer, facial cleanser, shampoo, conditioner, sunscreen, body wash, styling gel, acne treatments, foundation, eye shadow, mascara, baby wipes, hand cream, lubricant, hair spray, eye makeup remover. (It's also used as a preservative in food—and funeral homes!)

Why it's bad: Formaldehyde is harmful to the immune system, is a known human carcinogen, and has been linked to leukemia, irregular periods, asthma, Lou Gehrig's disease, and DNA damage.

NO: Parabens

Found in shampoo, conditioner, body wash, tooth whitener, toothpaste, facial cleanser, sunscreen, moisturizer, toners/astringents.

Why it's bad: Parabens have estrogenic effects on the body and are linked to breast and prostate cancer.

NO: Placenta

Found in some hair relaxers, moisturizers, and toners.

Why it's bad: Placenta can produce estrogen, estrone, estradiol, and progesterone, and increase your risk for breast cancer and other problems.

NO: Phthalates

Found in some nail polish, nail and cuticle treatments, fragrance, bath oil, moisturizer, and hair spray.

Why it's bad: Pthalates may be toxic to the reproductive system, causing infertility and birth defects. Because they're not listed on product labels, they can be hard to track down (sometimes hidden as "fragrance").

NO: Triclosan

Found in moisturizer, hand cream, shampoo, facial cleanser, conditioner, antiperspirant, exfoliant, body wash, toothpaste.

Why it's bad: Triclosan is believed to interfere with thyroid hormone metabolism, cause antibiotic resistance, and create carcinogenic compounds when combined with chlorinated water.

YES: Natural cosmetics and personal-care products

Some cosmetics claim to be "organic," but, unlike with food, no firm governmental guidelines for cosmetics or personal-care products exist. Until we have a reliable designation, check out Skin Deep, Environmental Working Group's cosmetics database (www.cosmeticsdatabase.com), which takes the ingredients in more than twenty-five thousand products and matches them with fifty toxicity and regulatory databases. It's amazing—you don't need to go anywhere else for information.

So many endocrine-disrupting chemicals are not yet regulated by the water authorities, and conventional water treatment methods are beyond ridiculous. (Check out your area's scorecard at the University of Cincinnati's database of metropolitan water sources at www.uc.edu/gissa/projects/drinkingwater/ or find your local water quality report from www.epa.gov/safewater/dwinfo/.)

The only way to get clean water is to use a water filter religiously. Once you have received your area's water report, find a filter that removes the contaminants at the National Science Foundation's complete database of verified brands of all types of water filters: www.nsf.org/Certified/dwtu. This quick chart will get you started. To be safest, combine two kinds of filters, such as reverse osmosis plus a faucet-mounted carbon filter.

Type	How Does It Work?	Pros	Cons
Reverse osmosis	Uses a semipermeable membrane to remove particles and molecules of dissolved contaminants	Removes all heavy metals, bacteria, viruses, and may remove some pharmaceuticals	Wasteful—creates 3 to 20 gallons of wasted water for every 1 gallon of usable water. Filters out all minerals, including healthful ones such as magnesium and potassium. Does NOT remove chlorine, pesticides, or herbicides. Some claim the water can be somewhat "flat" tasting.
Distilled	Brings water to a boil, then keeps temperature constant. Collects steam and condenses it back into water. (Impurities boil at higher temperatures so they can be easily collected and removed.)	Removes all heavy metals, bacteria, viruses	Wasteful—creates 5 gallons of wasted water for every 1 gallon of usable water. Filters out all minerals, including healthful ones such as selenium. Does NOT remove chlorine, pesticides, herbicides, or pharmaceuticals. Some claim the water can be somewhat "flat" tasting.

Type	How Does It Work?	Pros	Cons
Activated carbon filter (Standard 53-certified) (Comes in faucet-mount, under the sink, or in pitchers)	Water flows through a carbon filter that attracts and traps many impurities.	Vary by brand. All remove chlorine, improve taste, and reduce sediment. Most remove heavy metals and disinfection byproducts. Some remove parasites, pesticides, radon, and VOCs.	Does not filter out pharmaceuticals. Brands differ significantly on what contaminants they do and do not filter.

Here are some of my favorite natural cosmetic brands and how you can find them:

- Dr. Hauschka (www.drhauschka.com)
- Ren (www.renskincare.com)
- Aesops (www.aesop.net.au)
- Nude (www.nudeskincare.com)
- Jason (www.jasoncosmetics.com)

REMOVE TOXINS FROM YOUR HOUSE

According to the EPA, the air in your house could have one hundred times the level of pollutants in the air outside, primarily due to VOCs emitted from toxic cleaners and other household products. Try these tips to reduce your bioburden at home.

NO: Chemical home cleaners

Almost 90 percent of all poison exposures happen at home, most from items like cleaning supplies, medicines, cosmetics, and other personal-care items. The worst are drain, oven, and toilet bowl cleaners, and products containing chlorine or ammonia. (The combination of chlorine and ammonia creates a toxic chlorine gas, chloramine, used as a chemical weapon in World War I.)

YES: Use 100 percent natural products

Use truly natural products, such as white vinegar, hydrogen peroxide, lemon juice, and plain old water. No risk of endocrine disruption and a lot of bang for your buck!

I was terrified to realize how toxic some common household items are. Keep an eye out for these labels—check out just how dangerous they are! They're not talking about babies either—this is the amount that could drop a one-hundred-eight pound adult. Scary!

Poison, Danger, or Highly Toxic—If you swallow one teaspoon or less, you could die.

Warning or Very Toxic—If you swallow one teaspoon to one tablespoon, you could die.

Caution or Toxic—If you swallow one ounce to one pint, you could die.

White vinegar mixed with water can clean any kind of floor, window, mirror, or other shiny surface. Vinegar gets rid of stink in the sink and mold in the shower, cleans and softens clothes, and, when combined with baking soda, can unclog drains.

Castile soap and hot water clears away dirt—use it anywhere with baking soda and/or vinegar to get the job done.

Baking soda can be used to clean cutlery, deodorize stinky carpets and doggie couches, scrub toilets and tubs, and destink your fridge and freezer. Anyplace you once used scouring powder, you can use baking soda.

Lemon juice can be used as a substitute for bleach due to its whitening ability.

Hydrogen peroxide can be used, in combination with white vinegar, as one of the very best sanitizing kitchen cleansers. Susan Sumner, a food scientist at Virginia Polytechnic Institute and State University, created this process: Buy two empty spray bottles and fill one with hydrogen peroxide and the other with vinegar; spray your counter first with the vinegar, then with the hydrogen peroxide (or vice versa), and voilà! Tests proved this sequence of cleaning was more effective than any bleach-based cleanser at eliminating bacteria—and it doesn't emit bleach's cancerous dioxins. (Bonus: This spray also works on food—and after you rinse the food with water, it leaves no detectable residue.)

YES: Use reliably safe store-bought cleansers

Household cleaners that claim to be natural could be toxic and we'd never know. Stick with companies known to be environmentally responsible, such as Seventh Generation, Mrs. Meyer's, Dr. Bronner's, Ecover, and Method. Look for words like

ammonia-free
biodegradable

free of dye or perfume
noncarcinogenic
non–petroleum-based
nontoxic

NO: Artificial room deodorizers

These products only mask whatever foul odor is festering. They are little factories of VOCs just pumping toxins into your room.

YES: Clean your air with a HEPA filter

A study found that using HEPA filters for two days dramatically improved the cardiovascular function of healthy nonsmokers. Get one with a VOC filter.

YES: Surround yourself with green

NASA scientists found that one potted plant every one hundred square feet can remove many harmful contaminants from the air in your home. Best varieties include bamboo palm, English ivy, gerbera daisy, and green spider.

NO: Scotchgarded furniture or stain-resistant clothing

One PFC compound used to make stain-resistant fabrics and believed to cause birth defects and cancer was the most highly concentrated one in the breast milk of nursing mothers.

YES: Organic clothing whenever possible

Cotton farmers use the most (and most damaging) pesticides. Seek out organic cotton, especially for sheets and baby clothes.

▶ REMOVE TOXINS FROM YOUR YARD

Pesticides increase your risk of dozens of cancers, not to mention the virtual certainty of endocrine disruption and, eventually, insulin resistance. Getting the pesticides out of your home and your yard is pretty much job one.

DITCH YOUR DRY CLEANER

NO: Weed killer

Chemical lawn treatment companies use atrazine, a weed killer proven to cause extreme endocrine disruption. Boy frogs treated with atrazine look fine from the outside but grow girl parts on the inside—part of the reason frogs are dying out all over the world.

YES: Make your lawn organic

Mowing, watering, and fertilizing lawns contribute approximately 2 percent of America's fossil-fuel consumption and 10 percent of our air pollution. Check out www.safelawns.org for tons of useful tips.

YES: Plant a native garden

Beneficial bacteria found in soil could even help your brain produce more serotonin. One study found that the bacterium *Mycobacterium vaccae* activates pathways similar to the effects of antidepressant drugs.

REMOVE TOXINS FROM YOUR BABIES (PETS AND KIDS)

Taking care of babies and pets can bring a whole new layer of chemicals into your life. Protect them—and yourself—by making a few very conscious choices about their care.

NO: Pest-control shampoo

One recent study found that parents who'd bathed their pets with pyrethrin pest-control shampoos were twice as likely to have an autistic child.

YES: Natural pet shampoos

My pup Baxter and I alternate from Davines to Dr. Hauschka.

NO: Lice shampoo for kids

Every time you use lice shampoo, you're dumping pesticides on your kid's head.

YES: Adopt a "No nits!" policy

Use a lice comb and get the nits out before they develop into lice. Prevent recurrences with a few drops of tea tree essential oil sprinkled on their heads every day.

NO: Flame-retardant clothing

Make sure your kids' pajamas, bedding, pillows, and mattresses do not include polybrominated diphenyl ethers (PBDEs), chemicals linked to thyroid disruption, learning and memory problems, damage to hearing, decreased sperm counts, and birth defects.

YES: Organic bedding and clothing

Your body, your kids' bodies, and the planet will be much happier.

NO: Plastic toys

Many manufacturers and stores have pledged to remove phthalates from their toys, but if the recalls on toys from China tell us anything, it's that we can't be 100 percent sure of product claims.

YES: Wood and cloth toys

Choose unpainted wood and organic fabric toys, and do not buy toys made in China. (Sorry, but until they clean up their act, it's best to steer clear!)

NO: Soy formula

Unless your pediatrician says otherwise. Babies who drink soy formula consume a tremendous amount of phytoestrogens per pound of body weight.

YES: Breast-feed

Try to breast-feed, and if you can't, ask your pediatrician to recommend the best formula for your baby. Don't be scared that environmental toxins may leach into your breast milk. Experts say the benefits of breast-feeding surpass any potential dangers.

NO: BPA bottles or chlorine-bleached diapers

Don't put endocrine disruptors directly into your baby's mouth or on her bottom.

Choose glass bottles and unbleached diapers, such as Seventh Generation chlorine-free diapers or gDiapers.

▶ REMOVE TOXINS FROM YOUR MEDICINE CHEST

Now comes the big NO! Drugs.

Working with your doctor, I want you to remove all over-the-counter and prescription drugs whenever or wherever possible. Period. The end.

Look, I know I am taking a strong stance here. And ultimately, I wouldn't want to live in a world without modern medicine. But with rare exceptions, many pharmaceuticals create more problems than they solve.

Have you ever actually read the package insert that comes with your "medication"? It makes you wonder if the side effects of the drugs are more sinister than the existing condition.

The drugs you should be most mindful of are the ones I call the anti's: antidepressants, antiinflammatories, antibiotics, and so on. These drugs don't work with the body's natural biochemistry; they work against it. Except in extreme cases, their side effects can be much worse than the original condition: kidney stones, abnormal blood clotting, blood disorders, deafness, colitis, fungal infections, leaky gut, rash, difficulty breathing, nausea, diarrhea, inability to orgasm, anxiety, constipation, weight gain, sleep disruption, hair loss, raised blood pressure, anemia . . . the list goes on and on.

I have contestants come to the *Biggest Loser* campus while taking twelve different drugs. They start out with some type of obesity-related disease: high blood pressure, type-2 diabetes, arthritis, cholesterol, you name it. All these drugs have side effects. So their doctors write a prescription for another drug to treat the side effects. Within a month, the contestants are off those medications permanently. That's your miracle solution: diet and exercise.

Perhaps the scariest drugs—and the ones most antithetical to the Master Your Metabolism program—are synthetic hormones. Talk about endocrine disruptors! Women have been going through menopause for thousands of years. Suddenly, we think God/nature/evolution/(insert your personal belief system here) messed up? The drug companies turn around and sell us a disease that isn't a disease at all, and then they make a drug for it that kills us.

Think about what happened when the findings of the Women's Health Initiative, sponsored by the National Institutes of Health, came out in 2002. The eight-year study of estrogen-plus-progestin therapy was halted after five years, because the women on the study were dropping dead of heart attacks and strokes. The researchers analyzed the data and found that the combination of these synthetic hormones was responsible for a

- 26 percent higher incidence of breast cancer
- 22 percent increase in total cardiovascular disease
- 29 percent increase in heart attacks
- 41 percent increase in strokes
- 100 percent increase in the rate of blood clots in the lungs

Since those results were released, many women have backed off from HRT. But birth control pills are flying high, despite the National Toxicology Program's *Tenth Report on Carcinogens,* also published in 2002, which classified all steroidal estrogens—those used in HRT and birth control—to be carcinogens. The National Cancer Institute reports that while birth control pills decrease risks of ovarian and endometrial cancer, they also may increase risks of breast, cervical, and liver cancers.

Why isn't the FDA cracking down on this? Here's why: Pharmaceutical companies spend hundreds of millions of dollars to gain FDA approval for their products. Public funding can't keep up with the agency's expanding responsibilities, so more than 50 percent of the FDA's work checking safety and effectiveness is funded by the companies whose products are being reviewed. (Conflict of interest, you think?)

And on the other end of the pharmaceutical chain, the drug companies like to think the doctors work for them. They cater lunches and dinners for them and their entire staff. Doctors are required to do continuing education. Who do you think sponsors those costs for them? That's right: drug companies.

Now, certainly, not all doctors are bad. In fact, I work with many whom I would bow at their feet, they are so ethical, talented, and intelligent. In any profession you will have both good and bad.

So here is your best line of defense: Get checkups, practice preventive medicine, and be proactive. For the most part, you can reduce or even cure most ailments with diet and lifestyle changes. Use condoms for birth control. Eat well and live right to manage menopause naturally. Bottom line: Do your own research and get a second opinion, at the least, before taking a drug. Drugs have side effects. Exercise, food, and properly used vitamin supplements do not. Take drugs only as a last resort.

RESTORE LOST NUTRIENTS

Due to changes in farming methods, the sad state of our soil, and the lack of biodiversity in this country, even our whole food is not nearly as nutritious as it once was. And under constant assault from the environment we live in, our bodies need certain nutrients to help us cope properly with the toxicity. Considering all of this, it's not surprising that more than 80 percent of Americans are severely nutrient-deficient.

That's why after we Restore whole, nutritious foods to your diet, we must also Restore lost nutrients that you cannot get any other way, because certain missing vitamins and minerals are essential for hormone production. What you need, first and foremost, are a quality multivitamin, a calcium supplement, and a fish oil supplement.

No matter what brands you pick, try to find a multivitamin that includes the following key vitamins and nutrients, each essential for proper hormone function. I've listed the daily nutrient intakes recommended by the Linus Pauling Institute at Oregon State University, a world-renowned research center on the science of micronutrients. With a high-quality multi, calcium supplement, and fish oil capsule, combined with the Master diet, you should get to these levels quite easily.

BIOTIN: 30 mcg

People with type 2 diabetes who take biotin have lower fasting glucose levels. Biotin helps the body use more glucose to synthesize fatty acids. Biotin also stimulates glucokinase, a liver enzyme that increases glycogen synthesis and increases insulin release, which lowers blood glucose.

Food sources: 1 egg (25 mcg); 1 slice of whole wheat bread (6 mcg); 1 whole avocado (6 mcg)

FOLIC ACID: 400 mcg

One study showed that folic acid can help lower ACTH, an adrenal hormone that can lead to increased blood pressure. Ensuring adequate intake of folic acid is essential for any woman of childbearing age, even if you're not planning on getting pregnant—on the off-chance that you do, having folic acid in your body beforehand will prevent neural tube defects that result in brain and nervous system damage in babies.

Food sources: ½ cup cooked lentils (179 mcg); ½ cup cooked spinach (132 mcg); 6 spears asparagus (134 mcg)

NIACIN: 20 mg

Niacin protects your heart by increasing your HDL, lowering your LDL, and turning dangerous tiny LDL particles into larger, less heart-attack-inducing ones. Niacin may increase growth hormone release, but in people at risk for diabetes, large doses of niacin may cause a spike in insulin and triglycerides. Stick to the dosage in your multivitamin and you'll do great!

Food sources: 3 ounces tuna (11.3 mg); 3 ounces salmon (8.5 mg); 3 ounces turkey (5.8 mg)

PANTOTHENIC ACID: 5 mg

All steroid hormones, including estrogen and progesterone, as well as the neurotransmitter acetylcholine and melatonin, can only be produced when you have enough pantothenic acid, or vitamin B_5. Also, your liver needs vitamin B_5's coenzyme A to break down certain drugs and toxins.

Food sources: 1 whole avocado (2 mg); 8 ounces yogurt (1.35 mg); ½ cup sweet potato (0.88 mg)

RIBOFLAVIN: 1.7 mg

Riboflavin—aka vitamin B_2—helps metabolize vitamin B_6, niacin, and folic acid. Riboflavin is also involved in proper thyroid production and helps to control homocysteine levels.

Food sources: 1 cup nonfat milk (0.34 mg); 1 egg (0.27 mg); 3 ounces beef (0.16 mg)

THIAMINE: 1.5 mg

Thiamine helps metabolize glucose. Carb addicts are often deficient in thiamine. One study found that after four days of increasing carbohydrate intake, people's thiamine dropped up to 20 percent.

Food sources: 3 ounces lean cooked pork (0.72 mg); 1 cup long grain brown rice (0.21 mg); 1 ounce Brazil nuts (0.18 mg)

VITAMIN A: 2,500 IU

Vitamin A interacts with vitamin D and thyroid hormone to directly impact the way your genes are transcribed, helping teach each type of cell its specific job. Vitamin A also helps protect your immune system and your skin.

Food sources: ½ cup cooked butternut squash (1,907 IU); ½ cup chopped carrot (1,793 IU); ½ cup cooked collard greens (1,285 IU)

VITAMIN B$_6$: 2 mg

Vitamin B$_6$ helps the body release glucose from stored glycogen and synthesize the neurotransmitters serotonin, dopamine, and norepinephrine. Vitamin B$_6$ binds to the receptors for estrogen, progesterone, testosterone, and other steroid hormones, preventing the uptake of excessive hormones, which may help reduce the risk of breast and prostate cancer. Vitamin B$_6$ may also help relieve PMS, depression, and carpal tunnel syndrome caused by hypothyroidism.

Food sources: 3 ounces chicken (0.51 mg); 1 medium banana (0.43 mg); 6 ounces vegetable juice cocktail (0.26 mg)

COPPER: 900 mcg

Copper works with zinc to help maintain the thyroid, but an excess in one will create a deficiency in the other. Excess copper can also stimulate prostaglandin activity, interfere with antioxidants' activity, and lower your immune system, so stick to the dose in your multivitamin. Copper also helps dopamine convert into norepinephrine.

Food sources: 1 ounce cashews (629 mcg); 1 cup raw sliced mushrooms (344 mcg); 2 tablespoons peanut butter (185 mcg)

IRON: 18 mg*

Your body needs iron to properly use iodine to activate thyroxine. Researchers recently discovered a hormone called hepcidin, which regulates the iron levels in the body. If you have inflammatory bowel syndrome or other inflammation, you may have too much hepcidin and too little iron in your body. People with celiac disease, those who've had ulcers, vegetarians, and athletes are more prone to iron deficiencies.

Food sources: 6 medium oysters (5.04 mg); 1 tablespoon blackstrap molasses (3.5 mg): 3 ounces dark-meat chicken (1.13 mg)

MAGNESIUM: 320 mg (women)–420 (men) mg

Just a few days of magnesium deficiency may stimulate the release of inflammatory cytokines, pro-inflammatory molecules that are linked to insulin resistance. Between 25 and 38 percent of diabetics don't get enough magnesium, yet magnesium may help reduce blood glucose: People who eat more magnesium have a 30 percent lower chance of developing metabolic syndrome.

Food sources: 23 almonds (78 mg); ½ cup cooked Swiss chard (78 mg); ½ cup cooked lima beans (63 mg)

---

*Men and postmenopausal women rarely have deficiencies in iron, and too much can raise risks of heart disease; if you're in either group, seek out a multivitamin without iron for that reason. But premenopausal women, teens, and children all are at risk of iron deficiency and should supplement.

VITAMIN B$_{12}$: 30 mcg

Older people cannot absorb Vitamin B$_{12}$ from food and need supplements. Vegetarians must supplement with B$_{12}$ because we only get it from animal products. Diabetics are often B$_{12}$-deficient because the pancreas supplies the enzymes and calcium necessary to absorb B$_{12}$ from food.

Food sources: 3 ounces steamed clams (84 mcg); 3 ounces steamed mussels (20.4 mcg); 3 ounces cooked beef (2.1 mcg)

VITAMIN C: 400 mg

We can't make vitamin C, so we have to get it from our diets. Vitamin C is also important in helping to support the proper production of the adrenal hormones. Because your body cannot produce vitamin C, a bit more is usually a good idea in times of stress. People who take supplemental vitamin C on a regular basis may experience 25 to 40 percent lower risk of heart disease. Most supplements have only 60 mg, which is not enough to saturate your blood and cells—try to get to at least 400 mg with vitamin C–rich foods.

Food sources: ½ cup raw chopped sweet red pepper (141 mg); 1 cup strawberries (82 mg); 1 medium tomato (23 mg)

VITAMIN D: 2,000 IU*

Vitamin D helps the body regulate its calcium levels, boosts immunity, discourages autoimmune disorders (such as inflammation), lowers blood pressure, and may reduce the risk of osteoporosis and breast, colon, and prostate cancers. Too little vitamin D can negatively impact insulin and glucose levels in type 2 diabetics.

*Linus Pauling Institute also recommends ten to fifteen minutes of direct midday sun on arms and legs or face and arms at least three times a week.

Food sources: 3 ounces canned pink salmon (530 IU); 3 ounces canned sardines (231 IU); 8 ounces vitamin-D-fortified milk (98 IU)

VITAMIN E: 200 IU*

Vitamin E also helps slow the aging of cells and tissues and may help reduce the negative effects of environmental pollutants in the body. Lab studies have indicated that vitamin E may be especially effective in helping prevent and treat hormone-responsive cancers, such as breast and prostate.

Food sources: 1 ounce hazelnuts (4.3 mg); 1 tablespoon canola oil (2.4 mg); 1 tablespoon olive oil (1.9 mg)

VITAMIN K: 10 TO 20 mcg

Vitamin K helps the clotting of blood after injuries and protects against osteoporosis, kidney stones, cystic fibrosis, and—get this—body odor. Vitamin K is highly concentrated in the pancreas and may be involved in the healthy release of insulin after eating.

Food sources: 1 cup chopped raw kale (547 mcg); 1 cup raw spinach (299 mcg); 1 cup chopped raw broccoli (220 mcg)

ZINC: 15 mg

Zinc levels tend to be lower in older people, anorexics, alcoholics, people on crash diets, children with ADHD, and diabetics. Zinc levels are related to leptin, the hormone that helps us feel satisfied. Studies suggest that restoring deficiencies of zinc helps people increase lean body mass while maintaining or losing fat mass.

*The Linus Pauling Institute recommends 200 IU of *natural* d-alpha-tocopherol every day or 400 IU every other day.

Food sources: 6 medium oysters (76.3 mg); 3 ounces dark-meat turkey (3.8 mg); ½ cup baked beans (1.8 mg)

SELENIUM: 70 mcg

Most of the fat-burning T3 in our bodies is activated when selenium-dependent enzymes help convert T4 to T3 by removing one iodine atom. Selenium also produces other enzymes that help the body detox from the effects of environmental pollutants, pharmaceuticals, and radiation.

Food sources: 3 ounces crab meat (41 mcg); 3 ounces shrimp (34 mcg); 2 slices whole wheat bread (23 mcg)

CHROMIUM: 60–120 mcg

About 90 percent of us don't get enough chromium, but chromium helps insulin take glucose out of the blood and usher it into the cells. Low levels of chromium can lead to insulin dysfunction and high triglycerides, further increasing the risk of heart disease from people already predisposed to metabolic syndrome and cardiovascular trouble.

Food sources: ½ cup broccoli (11 mcg); 1 medium apple (1.4 mcg); ½ cup green beans (1.1 mcg)

POTASSIUM: 4.7 g

Potassium is both a mineral and an electrolyte that dances back and forth across the cell membrane, swapping sodium for potassium. This dynamic exchange of energy, which accounts for up to 40 percent of our resting metabolic rate, protects the cell membranes and is a key aspect of our nerve, muscle, and heart function.

Food sources: 1 medium baked potato (926 mg); ½ cup dried plums (637 mg); 6 ounces tomato juice (417 mg)

CALCIUM: 1,000–1,200 mg*

Calcium makes it possible for enzymes to break down glycogen, releasing energy for the muscles to use and preventing muscle cramps or spasms. Calcium also helps our nervous system send messages and plays a role in insulin secretion. Your body can only absorb 300 mg max at a time, so if you don't eat three servings of dairy a day, take your calcium supplements at two different times during the day.

Food sources: 1 cup yogurt (300 mg); ½ cup cooked Chinese cabbage (239 mg); ½ cup white beans (113 mg)

EPA AND DHA OMEGA-3 FATTY ACIDS: 1 g

Your body cannot make these fats, but you need them to survive. Fish oil capsules allow you to get the nearly miraculous health benefits without the heavy-metal toxicity and pesticide buildup in fish. Fish oil lowers triglycerides, blood pressure, LDL, inflammation, arterial plaque, and raises HDL, all of which help stave off heart disease. Fish oil also slashes the risk of death in those people already diagnosed with heart disease, by reducing prevalence of heart attacks, strokes, and abnormal heart rhythms. Burgeoning research suggests omega-3 supplementation can help prevent or treat other conditions, including ADHD, asthma, bipolar disorder, cancer, dementia, depression, and diabetes.

Food sources: 4 ounces wild-caught salmon (2 g); ¼ cup walnuts (2.27 g); 2 tablespoons flaxseeds (3.5 g)

> ## REBALANCE YOUR ENERGY OUT

You could follow this diet to the letter, get rid of all the toxins in your house, take the perfect vitamin supplements every day—but if you don't

---

*Your multivitamin likely has some calcium in it, but nowhere near the 1,000 to 1,200 mg of calcium that you need, because the pill wouldn't fit down your throat! Look for a calcium carbonate or calcium citrate supplement, as both are absorbed readily—carbonate is absorbed best with food, citrate without.

learn how to manage your stress and Rebalance your energy, you're still sabotaging your hormones.

We used to burn off our stress hormones cortisol and adrenaline when we outran lions in the jungle. Now, if our boss makes unreasonable demands, we can't release that stress by hauling off and popping him one. No, we just have to suck it up and sit there, with our hearts pounding and the adrenaline and cortisol pumping through our veins, and struggle to maintain our composure and be good and dutiful workers.

Constant overwork without adequate relaxation will keep your body in fight-or-flight mode for far too long, corroding your organs and glands until your system basically breaks down. People who secrete the most cortisol in response to stress also have the most fat on their bellies, no matter how much they weigh. They are also more likely to experience regular spikes in carb cravings.

When you overwork your brain and underwork your body, when you sleep too little and worry too much, your growth hormone levels don't get their regular daily and nightly bursts. You can't convert thyroid hormone as easily. Hunger hormone ghrelin shoots up; satiety hormone leptin plummets. Your blood sugar levels go through the roof, and within days, your body becomes insulin-resistant—*even if you're not overweight*.

I am all about hard work. But I believe in full recovery, as well. Let's look at how you can let your endocrine system take a breather, so it can repair itself and allow your hormones to Rebalance to their optimal levels again.

REBALANCE ENERGY TACTIC #1: SLEEP AT LEAST SEVEN HOURS A NIGHT

A full night's sleep is not a luxury—it is a basic necessity for healthy hormone balance. Once you dip below seven hours a night, you are at a much greater risk of diabetes, cancer, heart disease, stroke, depression—and many, many more pounds.

Some researchers believe that slow-wave sleep—the deep, dreamless sleep that you ideally sink into about three or four times a night—may actually regulate your metabolism. In fact, stage 4 slow-wave sleep, which begins about an hour after we fall asleep, is when we release our greatest pulses of growth hormone, the hormone that prompts the body to burn stored fat. When we're young, we spend about 20 percent of our sleep in slow-wave stages 3 and 4. But as we get older, we may only spend about 10 or even 5 percent there.

Sadly, just two nights of bad sleep will cut your satiety hormone leptin by 20 percent and increase your hunger ghrelin by 30 percent. That one-two punch makes you much more likely to snack on high-carb treats, which couldn't come at a worse time for your insulin levels—and a University of Chicago study found that just three nights of poor sleep makes your body 25 percent less sensitive to insulin, equivalent to the insulin resistance brought on by 20 to 30 extra pounds.

In order to block fat-storage hormones and allow the full release of fat-burning hormones, you need to get at least seven hours a night. Don't forget this one caveat:

Absolutely no carbs before bed. Your level of hunger hormone ghrelin needs to be high in order to slip into stage 3 or 4 sleep. Carbs depress ghrelin faster than any other nutrient, so eating anything, especially carbs, before bed can delay your entry into deeper sleep for several hours. The release of growth hormone is possible only when the body is in a semi-fasting state, so the insulin spike that comes after carbs will automatically interfere with growth hormone release. I am fanatical about restricting carbs before bed—why would you knowingly eat something that interferes with restorative sleep and blocks one of the most beneficial hormone releases of the entire day? Don't do it!

REBALANCE ENERGY TACTIC #2: MOVE YOUR BODY EVERY DAY

Exercise is the number one form of preventive medicine and dramatically affects your hormone balance. When you really put energy into it, exercise releases fat-burning growth hormone, reduces cortisol, and makes cells more sensitive to insulin. Intense exercise even increases your metabolism-boosting thyroid hormones for a brief time. And any type of exercise will boost testosterone.

Exercise also increases DHEA, which props up your burned-out adrenals to give you more energy, strengthen your libido, and help relieve depression. Exercise floods the body with endorphins, natural morphine-like biochemicals that cause the "runner's high." Endorphins improve your body's reaction to stress, enhance your mood, and even increase your pituitary's release of growth hormone.

To use exercise to balance your hormones, focus on these seven suggestions. (Note: If you're in the market for a step-by-step exercise program, I urge you to check out my first two books, *Winning By Losing,* for beginners, or *Making the Cut,* for intermediate to advanced.)

Get 4 to 5 hours a week. Forget that "walk across parking lots!" and "take the stairs!" fitness advice. You can't lose weight in ten-minute bursts of exercise. No, you need to get to the gym, work your ass off when you're there, and get the job done. You'll burn way more calories in less time and enjoy more hormonal benefits. Just three weeks of this level of exercise can start to reverse insulin resistance.

Go big. I want you sweating, stretching, pushing yourself. You should be reaching for 85 percent of your maximum heart rate (220 − your age = your maximum heart rate, or MHR). Intense exercise increases your body's release of endorphins and growth hormone.

Base your workout on strength training. Women who lift moderate to heavy weights produce more active growth hormone after their workouts, and for a longer timer, than women who do other kinds of exercise. The greater your muscle mass, the higher your metabolism and the more sensitive to insulin your muscles become. (This isn't limited to overweight people—average-weight people have much better hormone balance when they have more muscle.)

Use circuit training to combine cardio and weight training. Each of your five hours should be a combination of cardio and strength training. Circuit training does both. For example, do a set of squats, then immediately follow up with a set of pushups. Repeat each set three times, then move on to two other exercises that work two different parts of the body, and alternate those.

There. You're circuit training. It's that easy.

Try intervals, too. Do intervals of walking and running. Start by alternating thirty seconds of walking with thirty seconds of running. Do this for thirty minutes. Intervals give the same hormonal benefits and high excess postexercise oxygen consumption, or EPOC—also known as after-burn—as longer bouts of continuous intense exercise.

Add extra cardio *after* your first five hours. You can add on extra hours of cardio only *after* you do your circuit strength training. Try adding a thirty-minute-to-one-hour session in for a powerful two-a-day workout.

Do it even if you hate it. I do! But just like you work to pay the mortgage or your car payment, you do the work in the gym to protect your most important asset: a healthy body. Once you're on a steady path with exercise, you'll automatically feel less stress.

▶ REBALANCE ENERGY TACTIC #3: BE GOOD TO YOURSELF

Would you treat your kids the way you treat yourself? Would you want them to go without love, nurture, sleep, play? So why on earth would you treat yourself that way?

If I could burn one message into your brain permanently, it would be this: *Selfish* is not a four-letter word. Selfish does not mean narcissistic or conceited—it means healthy. I know from my own experience, and from watching thousands of people change their lives, that the only way to accomplish this is to put yourself first.

Detox your circle of friends. We have specific neurons in our brains that make us automatically reflect the emotions of the people around us. Ask yourself: Who makes me feel bad about myself when I hang out with them? Who leaves me feeling drained? Take steps to minimize any time you spend with that person.

Ask for help. No one gets anywhere in life without help. *Ask* for the promotion at work, *ask* the in-laws to watch the kids so you can fit in your yoga class, *ask* a trainer to teach you about exercise. One *Journal of the American Medical Association* study found that people who had a brief monthly chat with a coach—usually just ten to fifteen minutes—maintained more weight loss than people who didn't have any kind of personal contact with one.

Identify your sources of stress. When I lie awake at night with thoughts swimming around in my head, I get up and write them all down. I identify what is bothering me and I create a game plan to fix it.

Learn to meditate. Meditation is to the mind what exercise is to the body. It strengthens the prefrontal cortex, a part of your brain that regulates emotion. When that part of the brain becomes stronger, research shows that people tend to be happier and bounce back faster from negative events.

Try other forms of exercise. People who did tai chi and Qigong three times a week for twelve weeks significantly lowered their BMI, waist circumference, and blood pressure. The participants had high blood sugar at the beginning of the study, but after three months, their Hb1Ac, fasting insulin, and insulin resistance had all decreased.

Get a weekly massage. In a study of teenage girls with body image issues, those who'd received a massage had lower levels of anxiety, depression, and cortisol, and higher levels of dopamine, a neurotransmitter that enhances mood. Massage also elevates serotonin, the same action produced by many antidepressant medications.

Please take your vacations. Working more than forty hours a week doubles women's risk of depression and increases men's risk by 33 percent. But even with all this overtime, one out of every three of us doesn't take our allotted vacation time. Don't make yourself a sitting duck for a heart attack. You earned that vacation—take it.

Once you Rebalance your energy, all the pieces of the Master diet plan fall into place. You are armed with a program that will help your ability to manage stress—whether psychological or environmental. You have the knowledge that you need to steer clear of toxins that damage your metabolism. You know what foods to eat, and how to eat them, to trigger your fat-burning hormones and keep your fat-storage hormones low. In short, you have all the resources you need to handle any situation this crazy world can throw at you—and come out leaner, cleaner, and happier for it.

Let's turn now to the Master two-week meal plan and recipes—and you'll see how easy (and how delicious) the *Master Your Metabolism* eating plan can be.

THE MASTER MEAL PLANS AND RECIPES

The Meal Plans and 15-plus Quick and Easy Meals
to Get You In and Out of the Kitchen Fast

I know that learning a new way of eating can be a challenge. I want you to see how easy and incredibly satisfying it can be to eat the best way to optimize your hormones, without spending hours in the kitchen or millions of dollars at the store. That's why I put together sample menus and sixteen recipes that take all of the principles, Power Nutrient food groups, and strategies into account. Even if you decide you don't want to follow these to the letter, please just take a second to look them over. You'll be able to see very clearly how *Master Your Metabolism* looks in real life.

> ## MASTER YOUR FOOD MATH

Study after study shows us that the way to get all the benefits of all the nutrients is to eat whole foods in balance. These aren't just long-term benefits—after only four days on this type of diet, study participants felt more satisfied, burned more calories at rest and during exercise, burned more calories while they slept, improved their body composition, and burned more fat than those who followed a traditional diet.

When you eat the way your body wants you to eat, when you stay away

CHAPTER 9

it to a
you really
d or where it
all the right
er they use organics.
and ask them to prepare
your ed instead of fried. Blah, blah,
blah—w now all the right things to ask,
but the bottom line is that the quality of the
food probably isn't great. Restaurants are
businesses and they are out to make
money, so they are probably using cheap
ingredients like trans fats, HFCS,
nonorganic foods, and so on.

By cutting back on eating out, you will
save a fortune (money you can spend on
healthy groceries) and you will guarantee
your success of mastering your metabolism.

I do still eat out, but for no more than five
meals per week, and when I do, I order
white fishes or ocean-caught salmon,
healthy grains such as brown rice, and
plenty of vegetables. To stay on the plan, it's
that simple.

from endocrine-disrupting crap and eat whole, organic foods in the right ratios, your hormones naturally fall in line. Your insulin levels drop. Your cells get more sensitive to insulin and leptin. Your ghrelin levels stay down after meals. CCK rises. Your testosterone levels rise, burning fat and building muscle, even while you sleep. Your thyroid is primed and helps your metabolism continue to burn calories. Your estrogen levels stay in normal ranges. Your cortisol levels stay down, and your belly fat melts away.

You lose weight because you work with your hormones, not against them.

Now, how exactly do you do it? How do you put these foods together in the right ratios? Well, I'm going to make it easy for you.

From my previous writing on balancing your macronutrients, I realize that this can be confusing for people. (It was probably the thousands of e-mails I got from you that tipped me off.) Then, in my second book, I created menus and recipes to illustrate how to balance carbs, protein, and fat. Genius, right? I thought so. But you wanted it simpler and reminded me that not everyone is at home cooking meals all week long. Touché! In an effort to make this easy for you, I created Master Your Food Math. With this grab-and-go chart, all you have to do is simple arithmetic: 1 + 1 = a perfectly balanced, metabolism-firing meal. And you're out the door.

MASTER YOUR FOOD MATH: BREAKFAST

START WITH ONE OF THESE	THEN ADD ONE OF THESE
2 eggs	1 slice Ezekiel 4:9 bread (any variety)
4 egg whites	1 cup oatmeal
1 cup skim milk	1 cup Nature's Path 8-grain Synergy cereal

3 slices nitrate-free turkey bacon	½ fresh grapefruit
1 cup organic low-fat Greek yogurt	1 cup fresh organic mixed berries
1 cup low-fat cottage cheese	1 apple
2 slices organic nitrate-free ham	2 tomatoes, sliced
3 ounces nitrate-free all-natural lox	½ multigrain bagel
1 nitrate-free chicken sausage	1 cup buckwheat cereal
3 ounces grilled chicken	1 corn tortilla and unlimited salsa

MASTER YOUR FOOD MATH: LUNCH

START WITH ONE OF THESE	THEN ADD ONE OF THESE
5 ounces chicken breast (palm-sized)	1 serving baked corn chips and ⅛ avocado
5 ounces grilled lamb	½ cup brown rice
5 ounces baked halibut	1 small sweet potato
5 ounces seared tuna	½ cup quinoa
5 ounces flank steak	½ cup black beans
5 ounces baked tilapia	1 large artichoke
5 ounces grilled sea bass	½ cup brown rice pasta
5 ounces black cod	Unlimited tomato salad
5 ounces sirloin	½ cup white beans

MASTER YOUR FOOD MATH: AFTERNOON SNACK

START WITH ONE OF THESE	THEN ADD ONE OF THESE
½ cup hummus	Unlimited carrot sticks
20 raw walnuts	1 apple
1 Horizon low-fat mozzarella stick	10 Kashi 7-grain crackers
2 tablespoons organic almond butter	Unlimited celery sticks
3 slices organic turkey	1 Ezekiel multigrain tortilla
½ cup black bean dip	20 baked corn chips
1 cup low-sodium canned tuna packed in water	¼ avocado
1 cup organic yogurt	Unlimited blueberries
½ cup low-fat cottage cheese	2 slices watermelon

continued on the following page

(continued)

MASTER YOUR FOOD MATH: DINNER

START WITH ONE OF THESE	THEN ADD ONE OF THESE
4 ounces grilled salmon	Unlimited steamed broccoli
4 ounces marinated chicken breast	Unlimited leafy salad with raw broccoli and raw cucumber
5 large shrimp	1½ cups cooked carrots
5 ounces broiled pork chops	Unlimited roasted cauliflower
4 ounces grilled lamb chops	Unlimited steamed green beans
4 ounces turkey breast	Unlimited baked Brussels sprouts
5 ounces scallops	Unlimited steamed spinach
4 ounces Cornish hen	1 cup spaghetti squash
5 ounces mahimahi	Unlimited grilled mixed veggies

THE TWO-WEEK MEAL PLAN

This two-week meal plan is comprised of all the hormone health foods needed to get you ripped and keep you there. Each of these days was built using as many Power Nutrient food groups as possible. You will note that all the meals are balanced in fat, protein, and carbs, except dinner. Remember that dinner is predominantly protein and healthy fats with extremely high-fiber vegetables to keep your insulin levels low at night so that you can max out your growth hormone release while you sleep. This is also why there is no evening snack; I don't want any insulin in that body of yours after nine P.M.

The items in **bold** in the menus can be found in the Master Recipes. In the event you are not a recipe person, I've also incorporated some very simple grilled meat and steamed veggie dishes that are brainless and don't require a recipe. The answer to everyone's "What's for dinner?" problem is foil packets. Basically, you take your meat and your veggies, sprinkle on a capful of extra virgin olive oil and a dash of salt and pepper, wrap it up in some foil, toss it on the grill, and you are golden.

I've also compiled a shopping list to help get your kitchen stocked and get you amped—you'll find that on page 236, along with a list of my preferred brands of organic and natural foods.

HOW LONG SHOULD I GRILL IT?

I am not a whiz when it comes to cooking, but I can always depend on my grill to make me look good. For most people, meat cook times are a bit confusing at first. Don't sweat it—just follow this chart. Try to turn your meat only once, in the middle of the total cook time, to allow it to brown just right.

Meat	Grill Time
Burgers	5 to 8 minutes on each side (10 to 16 minutes total)
Chicken breast	4 to 6 minutes on each side (8 to 12 minutes total)
Fish (½-inch-thick fillet)	2 to 3 minutes on each side (4 to 6 minutes total)
Fish (1-inch-thick steak)	4 to 6 minutes on each side (8 to 12 minutes total)
Lamb chops	6 to 8 minutes on each side (12 to 16 minutes total)
Pork chops	6 to 8 minutes on each side (12 to 16 minutes total)
Pork tenderloin	6 to 9 minutes on each side (12 to 18 minutes total; keep turning meat)
Shrimp	3 to 4 minutes on each side (6 to 8 minutes total)
Steak	6 to 9 minutes on each side (12 to 18 minutes total)

MONDAY MEAL PLAN, DAY 1

MEAL	FOODS
Breakfast	Scrambled egg whites, fried tomatoes, and 1 grapefruit
Lunch	**Southwest Chicken Salad**
Snack	Orange with handful of walnuts
Dinner	Halibut skewers with eggplant, peppers, and onions

TUESDAY MEAL PLAN, DAY 2

MEAL	FOODS
Breakfast	**Berry Smoothie**
Lunch	Romaine lettuce salad with mixed raw veggies, balsamic vinegar and olive oil, and 5 large shrimp
Snack	Carrot sticks and hummus
Dinner	Wild Pacific salmon with grilled vegetables

WEDNESDAY MEAL PLAN, DAY 3

MEAL	FOODS
Breakfast	**Breakfast Burrito**
Lunch	**Ezekiel Penne with Almond Tomato Sauce** and 5 large grilled prawns
Snack	½ cup black beans and salsa
Dinner	Grilled pork chop with steamed green beans

THURSDAY MEAL PLAN, DAY 4

MEAL	FOODS
Breakfast	**Breakfast Parfait** with side of 2 scrambled egg whites
Lunch	Grilled chicken breast and steamed spinach with onions and mushrooms
Snack	Nonfat Greek yogurt with xylitol (natural sweetener), cinnamon, and crushed dry-roasted almonds
Dinner	**Chipotle Beef**

FRIDAY MEAL PLAN, DAY 5

MEAL	FOODS
Breakfast	3-egg-white omelet with tomatoes and sliced turkey breast and 1 piece Ezekiel 7-grain toast
Lunch	**Chicken Tacos with Drunken Beans**
Snack	Handful sunflower seeds
Dinner	**Lemon Garlic Shrimp with Veggies**

SATURDAY MEAL PLAN, DAY 6

MEAL	FOODS
Breakfast	**Healthy Eggs Benedict**
Lunch	**Hot Tuna Sandwich**
Snack	Organic low-fat mozzarella sticks and ½ cup blueberries
Dinner	Grilled tilapia with steamed cauliflower

SUNDAY MEAL PLAN, DAY 7

MEAL	FOODS
Breakfast	Buckwheat with skim milk and 2 scrambled egg whites
Lunch	Grilled tuna fillet with ¼ cup brown rice and mixed green salad
Snack	Carrot sticks and ½ cup hummus
Dinner	Pork tenderloin with steamed asparagus

MONDAY MEAL PLAN, DAY 8

MEAL	FOODS
Breakfast	3 egg whites, 1 turkey sausage, ½ Roma tomato, and 1 piece Ezekiel 7-grain toast
Lunch	½ cup black beans, ½ cup salsa, ¼ cup cheese, and 1 Ezekiel tortilla; ½ cup Greek yogurt for dipping
Snack	3 slices of watermelon with ¼ cup raw almonds
Dinner	Grilled flank steak with grilled onions and steamed Brussels sprouts

TUESDAY MEAL PLAN, DAY 9

MEAL	FOODS
Breakfast	1 packet Quaker instant oatmeal with 2 hard-boiled egg whites
Lunch	Sliced turkey breast and mixed veggies over romaine lettuce with oil and vinegar
Snack	Guiltless Gourmet baked corn chips with fresh salsa
Dinner	**Pepper Jack Cheeseburgers with Jalapeño Cumin Sauce** (at dinner use lettuce leaves instead of a bun)

WEDNESDAY MEAL PLAN, DAY 10

MEAL	FOODS
Breakfast	**Artichoke Scramble** with 1 piece Ezekiel 7-grain toast
Lunch	1 can Amy's Organic Medium Chili with Vegetables with small salad
Snack	Low-fat organic Cheddar with Kashi vegetable crackers
Dinner	Grilled salmon with **Mustard Lemon Braised Vegetables**

THURSDAY MEAL PLAN, DAY 11

MEAL	FOODS
Breakfast	1 serving Nature's Promise cereal with nonfat milk
Lunch	**Grilled Halibut Soft Tacos with Orange Salsa**
Snack	1 cup Amy's Organic Split Pea Soup
Dinner	Grilled chicken with grilled peppers and onions

FRIDAY MEAL PLAN, DAY 12

MEAL	FOODS
Breakfast	1 packet Quaker instant oatmeal, 1 cup blueberries, and 2 scrambled egg whites
Lunch	**Quinoa-Stuffed Artichokes** with side of turkey breast
Snack	1 cup mixed berries with ¼ cup pecans
Dinner	Poached wild-Pacific salmon with blanched broccoli, carrots, onions, and celery

SATURDAY MEAL PLAN, DAY 13

MEAL	FOODS
Breakfast	3-egg-white omelet with green pepper and tomato and 1 slice Ezekiel bread
Lunch	5 large prawns with mixed greens and raw veggies with Galeos Caesar salad dressing
Snack	5 slices organic turkey with 1 peach
Dinner	**Roasted Garlic Chicken with Green Beans Amande**

SUNDAY MEAL PLAN, DAY 14

MEAL	FOODS
Breakfast	1 packet Quaker instant oatmeal and 1 cup Greek yogurt with 1 cup strawberries
Lunch	½ cup refried beans, shredded romaine, chopped onions, and tomatoes in 1 Ezekiel tortilla
Snack	1 apple with almond butter smeared on top
Dinner	Seared tuna steak with a mixed green salad

If you've taken a look at the Master Meal Plan, you no doubt already know that this diet is a snap. I tried to take all the guesswork out of cooking, so all you have to do is pull up a chair and enjoy. To design these recipes, I worked with Cassandra Corum, an organic chef, who helped me interpret the principles of this diet into delicious meals that trigger weight-loss hormones. Each one takes the very best, freshest whole foods and turns them into hormonally active, metabolic powerhouses—but all you'll taste is mouthwatering deliciousness. Enjoy!

RECIPE INDEX

ARTICHOKE SCRAMBLE
(Day 10 Breakfast)
Serves 4

4 medium-large artichokes
Nonfat cooking spray
3 teaspoons minced shallots
Salt to taste
8 medium egg whites
1 teaspoon lemon juice
2 to 3 sprigs parsley, minced, for garnish

Preheat the oven to 425° F.

Cut out the hearts from the artichokes and place them on a lightly greased baking sheet. Cook in the oven for 10 to 15 minutes or until soft and done.

Coat a medium sauté pan with nonstick cooking spray, then add the shallots and a dash of salt. Lightly sweat the shallots, then add the egg whites to the pan and scramble together. Remove from the heat, then add the lemon juice.

Place the eggs on top of the artichoke hearts, and serve garnished with minced parsley, if desired.

Per serving: Calories: 95.8, Cholesterol: 0 mg, Fat: 0.3 g, Saturated fat: 0 g, Calories from fat: 5.4, Trans fat: 0 g, Protein: 11.6 g, Carbohydrates: 14.8 g, Sodium: 231.7 mg, Fiber: 7 g, Sugars: 1.8 g

BERRY SMOOTHIE
(Day 2 Breakfast)
Serves 4

1 cup reduced-fat or fat-free milk
1 cup plain Greek yogurt
1½ cups frozen blueberries
1½ cups frozen strawberries
¾ cup ice
2 tablespoons flaxseed
¼ cup applesauce
1 tablespoon honey *or* 1 packet Stevia extract

Place all ingredients in a blender, and mix until smooth. Pour into glass and serve.

Per serving: Calories: 193.5, Cholesterol: 2.4 mg, Fat: 4.1 g, Saturated fat: 0.5 g, Calories from fat: 16.4, Trans fat: 0 g, Protein: 8 g, Carbohydrates: 34 g, Sodium: 87 mg, Fiber: 6.6 g, Sugars: 21 g

BREAKFAST BURRITO
(Day 3 Breakfast)
Serves 4

Nonstick cooking spray
1 large garlic clove, minced
3 cups prewashed spinach
8 large egg whites
Crushed red pepper to taste
Four 6-inch Ezekiel tortillas, warmed
3 large Roma tomatoes, chopped
½ cup grated nonfat pepper jack cheese

Lightly coat a medium skillet with nonstick cooking spray. Heat on medium, add garlic, and cook until fragrant. Add in spinach and cook until soft.

Coat a separate skillet lightly with cooking spray and scramble the egg whites. When almost finished, sprinkle in a moderate amount of crushed red pepper, depending on your taste.

Place equal amounts of spinach and egg in each tortilla, top with tomatoes and cheese, and serve.

Per serving: Calories: 400.3, Cholesterol: 6.3 mg, Fat: 9.4 g, Saturated fat: 3 g, Calories from fat: 32, Trans fat: 0 g, Protein: 27.5 g, Carbohydrates: 54.3 g, Sodium: 951 mg, Fiber: 8 g, Sugars: 6.5 g

BREAKFAST PARFAIT
(Day 4 Breakfast)
Serves 4

1 cup plain fat-free Greek yogurt
2 cups Nature's Path flax cereal
1 cup fresh blueberries or defrosted frozen blueberries
1 cup fresh or defrosted strawberries
4 teaspoons pure honey
1 medium-large orange, peeled and thinly sliced

In 4 small bowls or large cups, place ⅛ of a cup of yogurt to line the bottom. Layer ½ cup cereal, ¼ cup of each berry, and 1 teaspoon of honey. Cover with another layer of yogurt, and top with 2 to 3 orange slices. Serve cold.

Per serving: Calories: 165.8, Cholesterol: 3.6 mg, Fat: 2 g, Saturated fat: 0.6 g, Calories from fat: 10.2, Trans fat: 0 g, Protein: 6.2 g, Carbohydrates: 34.7 g, Sodium: 106.6 mg, Fiber: 6.5 g, Sugars: 21.9 g

HEALTHY EGGS BENEDICT
(Day 6 Breakfast)
Serves 4

Nonstick light cooking spray
3 cloves garlic, minced
1 10-ounce bag prewashed spinach (washed again)
Salt to taste
2 quarts water
3 ounces white vinegar
4 large eggs
2 large red tomatoes, sliced
4 multigrain English muffins, toasted
Freshly ground black pepper to taste

Coat a medium sauté pan with nonstick cooking spray and heat on medium. Heat garlic until slightly tender, add the spinach, and cook until soft, adding a pinch of salt if desired.

Bring the water and vinegar to a slow boil in a medium saucepan. Crack open an egg in a small bowl or cup to ensure that there aren't any pieces of shell in the yolk or white. With a wooden spoon, quickly stir the liquid in the pot to create a spiral, or "tornado," gently pour the egg into the center of the tornado, and stop stirring. Remove the egg with a slotted spoon when it looks like it has cooked through. Repeat with the remaining 3 eggs.

Place tomato slices on toasted muffin halves, followed by the desired amount of spinach, and top with egg and black pepper to taste. Serve.

Per serving: Calories: 266.6, Cholesterol: 211 mg, Fat: 6.7 g, Saturated fat: 1.8 g, Calories from fat: 16.2, Trans fat: 0 g, Protein: 15.2 g, Carbohydrates: 37.9 g, Sodium: 483 mg, Fiber: 4.5 g, Sugars: 3.6 g

CHICKEN TACOS WITH DRUNKEN BEANS

(Day 5 Lunch)

Serves 4

4 large boneless, skinless chicken breasts

Kosher salt to taste

Freshly ground black pepper to taste

Nonstick cooking spray

3 medium slices nitrate-free turkey bacon

1 clove garlic, minced

2 medium fresh jalapeños, minced

1 large can (16 ounces) refried black beans

1 small can (14.5 ounces) low-sodium 99 percent fat-free chicken broth

1 bottle light beer, preferably Corona Light

1 cup shredded romaine lettuce

1 cup chopped Roma tomatoes

4 6-inch Ezekiel tortillas

Dust the chicken with kosher salt and pepper. Place on a preheated grill and cook until done. Chop, and set aside.

Lightly coat a medium skillet with nonstick cooking spray. Lightly brown the bacon. Add the garlic and jalapeños, and sauté until the garlic is soft and fragrant, 1 to 2 minutes. Add the beans, then slowly add the broth, stirring until smooth. Use half the can of broth, as the beer will bring the beans to the desired consistency. Slowly stir in the beer. Spoon chopped chicken into 4 tortillas. Serve the beans next to the tacos, shredded romaine, and tomatoes.

Per serving: Calories: 150, Cholesterol: 49.9 mg, Fat: 1.8 g, Saturated fat: 0.4 g, Calories from fat: 13, Trans fat: 0 g, Protein: 21.8 g, Carbohydrates: 6.6 g, Sodium: 452 mg, Fiber: 2.5 g, Sugars: 3 g

EZEKIEL PENNE WITH ALMOND TOMATO SAUCE

(Day 3 Lunch)

Serves 4

2 cups Ezekiel penne pasta

2 cups tomato sauce

¼ teaspoon crushed red pepper flakes

¼ teaspoon kosher salt

8 large basil leaves

1½ tablespoons dry-roasted unsalted almonds, finely chopped

Freshly grated Parmesan cheese (optional)

Cook the pasta according to the package instructions. Set aside briefly.

In a large mixing bowl or blender, mix the tomato sauce, crushed red pepper, salt, basil, and almonds until smooth and combined. Place the pasta in bowls and top with the sauce and cheese, if using. Serve immediately.

Per serving: Calories: 312, Cholesterol: 52 mg, Fat: 5.3 g, Saturated fat: 0.7 g, Calories from fat: 26.4, Trans fat: 0 g, Protein: 11.3 g, Carbohydrates: 56.5 g, Sodium: 670.7 mg, Fiber: 2.1 g, Sugars: 10 g

GRILLED HALIBUT SOFT TACOS WITH ORANGE SALSA

(Day 11 Lunch)

Serves 4

TACOS

1 tablespoon extra virgin olive oil

1 tablespoon ancho chile powder

1 teaspoon freshly squeezed lime juice

¼ teaspoon kosher salt

⅛ teaspoon freshly ground black pepper

Four 4- to 6-ounce halibut fillets, 1 inch thick, skin on

Eight 6-inch corn tortillas

SALSA

2 large oranges

2 medium limes

1 teaspoon finely chopped cilantro

½ clove garlic, minced

2 teaspoons rice wine vinegar

Salt and pepper to taste

1 medium serrano chile, minced

1 tablespoon extra virgin olive oil

FOR THE TACOS:

In a large Ziploc bag, combine the oil, chile powder, lime juice, salt, pepper, and fillets. Shake the mixture until the fillets are fully coated.

Place the fillets on a preheated grill, skin side down, and grill until cooked through.

Remove the skin from the fillets and separate equally among the tortillas.

FOR THE SALSA:

Peel the oranges and limes, removing all the membranes (use just the juicy meat). Finely chop the fruit.

Mix together the fruit, cilantro, garlic, vinegar, salt, pepper, oil, and the serrano chile. Set aside.

Top the tacos with salsa and serve.

Per serving: Calories: 306.2, Cholesterol: 75 mg, Fat: 8 g, Saturated fat: 1.2 g, Calories from fat: 16.3, Trans fat: 0 g, Protein: 25.9 g, Carbohydrates: 36.3 g, Sodium: 93.3 mg, Fiber: 5.4 g, Sugars: 7.1 g

HOT TUNA SANDWICH

(Day 6 Lunch)

Serves 4

Nonstick cooking spray

¼ cup chopped onion

½ tablespoon minced garlic

Salt to taste

2 cans albacore tuna in water

½ teaspoon crushed red pepper

2 tablespoons whole grain mustard

4 slices multigrain bread, toasted

Lightly coat a medium skillet with nonstick cooking spray and heat over medium-high heat.

Add the onion, garlic, and a dash of salt. Stirring frequently, cook for 1 to 2 minutes. Add the tuna and the crushed red pepper, mix completely with the onions and garlic, and heat.

Spread ½ tablespoon whole grain mustard on each slice of toast, then spoon the tuna mixture over each slice and serve.

Per serving: Calories: 174, Cholesterol: 24.8 mg, Fat: 1.9 g, Saturated fat: 0.4 g, Calories from fat: 9.4, Trans fat: 0 g, Protein: 24.8 g, Carbohydrates: 13.3 g, Sodium: 151.4 mg, Fiber: 2.2 g, Sugars: 2.3 g

QUINOA-STUFFED ARTICHOKES

(Day 12 Lunch)

Serves 4

4 large artichokes

1 cup quinoa, uncooked

2 cups water

¼ cup sun-dried tomatoes

1 teaspoon kosher salt

1 teaspoon freshly ground black pepper

1 large lemon

ARTICHOKE PREP:

Boil the artichokes until tender.

Cut off the top inch of each artichoke, as well as the stem. Peel off the outer tough leaves and cut away all spiky edges. Separate the outer leaves to loosen them, as well as the inside leaves to make the lighter leaves around the heart visible. Pull out the lighter-colored leaves and remove the choke with a spoon.

FOR THE STUFFING:

Bring the quinoa and water to a boil, reduce the heat, and simmer until the water is soaked up and the quinoa is soft.

Stir in the sun-dried tomatoes, salt, and pepper, then squeeze the juice from the lemon onto the quinoa. Mix.

Preheat the oven to 375° F.

Scoop ¼ to ½ cup quinoa stuffing into each artichoke and around the sides in the gaps in the leaves.

Place in the oven to heat for 5 to 8 minutes. Serve.

Per serving: Calories: 344.9, Cholesterol: 0 mg, Fat: 4.4 g, Saturated fat: 0.6 g, Calories from fat: 30.2, Trans fat: 0 g, Protein: 16.3 g, Carbohydrates: 66.7 g, Sodium: 470.5 mg, Fiber: 15.7 g, Sugars: 7.8 g

SOUTHWEST CHICKEN SALAD

(Day 1 Lunch)

Serves 4

½ cup lime juice

2 tablespoons olive oil

4 medium garlic cloves, minced

8 tablespoons chopped cilantro
1 to 2 teaspoons chile powder
1 to 2 teaspoons ground cumin
1 teaspoon salt (optional)
Nonstick cooking spray
4 medium boneless, skinless chicken breasts
One 15-ounce can black beans, drained
4 medium-large Roma tomatoes, diced
8 tablespoons chopped scallions
4 cups organic romaine lettuce

Place the lime juice, olive oil, garlic, cilantro, chile powder, cumin, and salt (if using) in a closed jar. Shake until well mixed.

Lightly coat a grill with nonstick cooking spray, heat, and grill the chicken until done. Slice into 1-inch strips.

Mix together the chicken, beans, tomatoes, scallions, lettuce, and jar mixture, and serve.

Per serving: Calories: 415.3, Cholesterol: 68.4 mg, Fat: 11 g, Saturated fat: 1.7 g, Calories from fat: 35.9, Trans fat: 0 g, Protein: 41.2 g, Carbohydrates: 42.7 g, Sodium: 129.7 mg, Fiber: 16.7 g, Sugars: 8.3 g

DINNERS

CHIPOTLE BEEF
(Day 4 Dinner)
Serves 4

2½ to 3 pounds chuck roast
Kosher salt to taste
Freshly ground black pepper to taste
Nonstick cooking spray
1 can (15 ounces) low-sodium beef broth
1 can (7 ounces) chipotle peppers in adobe sauce
2 bags prewashed salad lettuce of your choosing

Dust the meat with salt and pepper. Coat a medium skillet with nonstick cooking spray. Heat the pan over medium-high heat, then brown the meat on both sides.

Add the broth and the entire contents of the can of chipotle peppers, sauce included.

Cook over low heat for 1 to 2 hours, then slice and serve over lettuce for a delicious spicy salad that doesn't need dressing.

Per serving: Calories: 457.2, Cholesterol: 170.1 mg, Fat: 20.3 g, Saturated fat: 7.8 g, Calories from fat: 41, Trans fat: 0 g, Protein: 62 g, Carbohydrates: 2.5 g, Sodium: 961.9 mg, Fiber: 0.7 g, Sugars: 0.6 g

LEMON GARLIC SHRIMP WITH VEGGIES
(Day 5 Dinner)
Serves 4

Nonstick cooking spray

1 large red bell pepper, diced

1 large green bell pepper, diced

2 pounds asparagus, trimmed and cut into 1- to 2-inch lengths

2 teaspoons minced lemon zest

½ teaspoon salt

6 cloves garlic, minced

1 pound raw shrimp, peeled and deveined

1 teaspoon cornstarch

1 cup non—reduced sodium chicken broth

1 tablespoon fresh lemon juice

2 tablespoons chopped parsley

Coat a medium skillet with nonstick cooking spray, and heat over medium. Add the bell peppers, asparagus, lemon zest, and ¼ teaspoon salt. Stir occasionally. When the vegetables just begin to soften, transfer to a bowl and cover.

Add remaining ¼ teaspoon salt to the skillet with the garlic, and sweat about 1 minute. Add the shrimp and cook for another 1 to 2 minutes.

Whisk the cornstarch and broth in a separate bowl until smooth, then add to the pan along with a dash of salt. Cook, stirring, until the sauce has thickened slightly and the shrimp are pink and just cooked through, about 2 to 3 minutes. Remove from the heat and stir in the lemon juice.

Serve the shrimp over the vegetables and garnish with parsley.

Per serving: Calories: 187.2, Cholesterol: 172.4 mg, Fat: 4.8 g, Saturated fat: 0.8 g, Calories from fat: 16.5, Trans fat: 0 g, Protein: 25.7 g, Carbohydrates: 10.9 g, Sodium: 176.8 mg, Fiber: 3.2 g, Sugars: 3.4 g

MUSTARD LEMON BRAISED VEGETABLES
(Day 10 Dinner)
Serves 4

1 tablespoon olive oil

2 pounds mixed vegetables

¼ cup chopped white onion

1 teaspoon salt

⅔ cup low-sodium chicken broth

2 teaspoons lemon juice

2 teaspoon Dijon mustard

Heat oil in medium skillet. When hot, add vegetables and a dash of salt. Stir frequently until vegetables start to soften and brown, about 3 to 5 minutes.

Slowly pour in chicken broth, cover, and simmer until broth has been absorbed and evaporated.

Uncover, add lemon juice and mustard, and combine with vegetables. Season to taste with remaining salt. Serve.

Per serving: Calories: 193, Cholesterol: 0 mg, Fat: 5.284 g, Saturated fat: 0.824 g, Calories from fat: 3.62, Trans fat: 0 g, Protein: 8.636 g, Carbohydrates: 32.757 g, Sodium: 631.69 mg, Fiber: 9.42 g, Sugars: 0.77 g

PEPPER JACK CHEESEBURGERS WITH JALAPEÑO CUMIN SAUCE
(Day 9 Dinner)
Serves 4

3 large fresh jalapeños, seeded and coarsely chopped

½ cup plus 3 tablespoons coarsely chopped cilantro

3 large garlic cloves, smashed

1 tablespoon fresh lime juice

1 teaspoon cumin

2 tablespoons water

Pinch of kosher salt

1½ pounds ground grass-fed lean sirloin, at room temperature

4 ounces nonfat pepper jack cheese, shredded

Freshly ground black pepper to taste

Olive oil, for brushing

4 regular multigrain or Ezekiel hamburger buns (just the bottoms)
1 cup shredded romaine lettuce
4 thin tomato slices
Sliced pickled jalapeños, for serving

In a blender, combine the jalapeños with ½ cup cilantro, the garlic, lime juice, ½ teaspoon of the ground cumin, water, and a pinch of salt. Puree until smooth.

In a medium bowl, lightly knead the sirloin with the pepper jack cheese, the remaining cilantro, and the remaining ½ teaspoon of cumin. Loosely shape into 4 patties about ¾ of an inch thick, and tuck any large pieces of cheese into the burgers.

Season with salt and pepper and transfer to a plate lined with plastic wrap.

Brush the grate of a hot grill with a little olive oil. Grill the burgers for about 10 minutes, turning once, over medium heat. Set the burgers on the buns and top with the lettuce, tomato, and jalapeño slices. Serve.

Per serving: Calories: 427, Cholesterol: 103.5 mg, Fat: 13.9 g, Saturated fat: 4.8 g, Calories from fat: 34.3, Trans fat: 0 g, Protein: 56 g, Carbohydrates: 18 g, Sodium: 714 mg, Fiber: 2.8 g, Sugars: 5.8 g

ROASTED GARLIC CHICKEN WITH GREEN BEANS AMANDE
(Day 13 Dinner)
Serves 4

CHICKEN
1 teaspoon olive oil
Kosher salt to taste
Freshly ground black pepper to taste
1 head garlic
4 large boneless, skinless chicken breasts

GREEN BEANS
1 cup green beans, washed and trimmed
Nonstick cooking spray
2 cloves garlic, minced
1 tablespoon raw almonds, sliced

FOR THE CHICKEN:

Preheat the oven to 375° F.

Drizzle the olive oil and a pinch of salt and pepper over the garlic head, and wrap it in aluminum foil. Roast the garlic about 15 to 20 minutes, until it is halfway done.

While the garlic is roasting, lightly dust the chicken breasts with salt and pepper.

Remove the garlic from the oven, then carefully pinch out the garlic cloves onto the chicken. Put the chicken on a roasting rack and place in the oven. Cook for 18 to 20 minutes.

FOR THE GREEN BEANS:

Bring 2 quarts of salted water to a boil. Place the green beans in the water for 2 to 3 minutes. Remove and pat dry.

Lightly coat a medium saucepan with nonstick cooking spray. Heat the pan on medium, then add the minced garlic and the almonds. Cook until the almonds turn slightly brown. Add the green beans and cook until combined and hot.

Serve with the chicken.

Per serving: Calories: 308.8, Cholesterol: 37.8 mg, Fat: 18.4 g, Saturated fat: 3.6 g, Calories from fat: 27.5, Trans fat: 0 g, Protein: 15.7 g, Carbohydrates: 21 g, Sodium: 397.3 mg, Fiber: 3.7 g, Sugars: 1.4 g

CHAPTER 10

THE MASTER REMEDIES

PROGRAMS FOR 6 OF THE MOST COMMON
HORMONAL DISORDERS

I designed *Master Your Metabolism* for everyone—whether you're young, old, male, female, thin, or packing a few extra pounds, the program will work for you. However, there are some times when all of your hormones go a bit further south, such as at menopause and andropause. When you have a more complex hormonal condition, such as PCOS, metabolic syndrome, PMS, or a thyroid imbalance, this diet will certainly help. But you may need a little extra help, support, and, possibly, medication.

I've been lucky enough to work with one of the nation's leading endocrinologists, Dr. Christine Darwin, an associate professor of medicine and associate chief for clinical research, clinical epidemiology, and preventive medicine at the UCLA Medical Center. She's helped me create programs that, along with this diet, can help you find some relief for these conditions.

> ### MASTERING PMS

Premenstrual syndrome, or PMS, is a little slice of hell on earth. Up to 75 percent of women experience this constellation of unpleasant symptoms that rise during the second half of their cycle, usually five to seven

217

days before their period. Just look at the number of symptoms often cited in connection with PMS:

Acne	Dizziness	Mood swings
Aggression	Faster or more pronounced	Muscle tension
Anxiety	heartbeat	Nausea
Bloating	Fatigue	Paranoia
Constipation	Feeling overwhelmed	Prickly hands and feet
Cramps and pressure in	"Foggy" thinking	Quick temper
the lower belly	Forgetfulness	Sensitivity
Cravings	Headaches	Swollen hands and feet
Crying	Hot flashes	Teary
Depression	Insomnia	Tender breasts
Desire to be left alone	Irritability	Vomiting
Distractibility	Loss of libido	Weight gain

Many women have several of these symptoms; some may have only one or two. One in twenty women experience such severe PMS that it can actually be considered premenstrual dysphoric disorder (PMDD), a potentially life-destroying condition, one of the symptoms of which can be uncontrollable anger. (If your PMS interferes with your normal functioning at work, home, or with loved ones, take it seriously and talk to your doctor.)

The true cause of PMS is a source of much controversy among endocrinologists. Many physicians blame the rapid rise and fall in progesterone levels after ovulation. Other physicians blame androgen disorders. Many experts believe PMDD may be caused by lower levels of serotonin, the calming "good mood" neurotransmitter. Thyroid disorders share many of the same symptoms as PMS—if you have chronic PMS, you might consider asking your doctor for a thyroid test, to rule out any problems there.

The good news is that PMS can be tamed if not cured. Make a note on your calendar on the first day of your period and track how many days you have in your cycle. Do this for three months, and patterns will emerge. Once you know what to expect, you can take direct steps to manage your own symptoms. Try these five tips:

Rest, relax, and exercise. Adequate sleep and less stress will put you in a better hormonal position to handle this physiological imbalance. You may not want to, but get in your workout anyway. The endorphin rush will help relieve cramps and counterbalance a likely dearth of serotonin and happy neurochemicals.

If you can, schedule around your period. Try to schedule downtime into the last and first weeks of your cycle—that's when PMS and then your period hit. Schedule stressful tasks for the second week of your cycle, which starts seven days after the first day of your period, because several hormones, such as LH, estrogen, and testosterone, not to mention your energy and focus, peak during this week before ovulation.

Cut out most caffeine, alcohol, and salt. Women with fibrocycstic breasts often experience a lot of tenderness during the premenstrual days. Reducing caffeine can minimize breast tenderness as well as irritability. Steer clear of alcohol, as it exacerbates feelings of depression. Cutting salt will reduce bloat.

Minimize simple sugars. Eating high-glycemic carbs increases the level of inflammation in your body, making cramps worse. A blood sugar roller coaster is never a good thing for your already raw nerves, so this diet gives you regular meals and snacks with fiber and protein to help keep that blood sugar stable.

Supplement. Calcium can reduce symptoms of PMS—shoot for at least 1,200 milligrams a day, a dose shown to be effective versus placebo in clinical trials on PMS. Magnesium is also helpful, as are B complex vitamins, with B_1, B_2, B_3, and especially B_6. To reduce the inflammation of cramps and breast tenderness, try a primrose oil supplement, a nonsteroidal anti-inflammatory that may work in ways similar to ibuprofen.

▶ MASTERING HYPOTHYROID

An underactive thyroid is death to your metabolism and can make attempts at weight loss very frustrating. Yet hypothyroidism, or low thyroid function, becomes increasingly common as women get older—up to one in five can experience some form, especially those who are white or Mexican-American. Check out the list of symptoms on page 41 and ask yourself if you've experienced one or more—but realize that sometimes you could have none of these symptoms and still be hypothyroid.

The most common cause of hypothyroid is Hashimoto's disease, an autoimmune condition in which the immune system attacks and damages the thyroid, impairing your ability to make thyroid hormones. Concern is growing that a great deal of hypothyroidism is being caused by environmental pollution and the release of pesticide buildup from our fatty tissues. Sometimes a less-than-thriving thyroid actually has more to do with your stress level and adrenal function than with the thyroid itself. Adrenal hormones, such as cortisol, play a big part in proper thyroid function; high levels can hinder conversion of T4 into T3. To rule out this stress-induced hypothyroidism, ask your doctor to run a test for ACTH and cortisol at the same time as your TSH test for thyroid function. (See chapter 2 for more information on thyroid testing.)

If your test indicates hypothyroidism, seek out an endocrinologist—they have experience with the subtleties of thyroid dysfunction. Try to find one who is open to solutions beyond thyroid medication, especially nutritional and lifestyle strategies to manage your thyroid. (Check out the "Find an Endocrinologist" search tool at The Hormone Foundation Web site, www.hormone.org/FindAnEndo/index.cfm.) If you are diagnosed with low thyroid function, try the following steps:

Follow the Master diet—with a few modifications. The program eliminates many of the environmental and nutritional toxins that have been shown to create thyroid problems. Do take care to cook goitrogenic cruciferous veggies, though—they're known to stimulate goiters. Also, don't take a multivitamin with iron or a cholesterol-lowering medication, or eat anything with iron, calcium, soy, or high fiber, within a few hours of your thyroid medication—these can all interfere with thyroid hormone absorption.

Exercise and relax every day. The stress hormone cortisol interferes with the conversion of inactive T4 hormone to the active T3 form. Exercise is a great stress reliever that lowers cortisol levels while also increasing your body's sensitivity to thyroid hormones. Check out some of the other relaxation recommendations in chapter 8 and, as a general rule, shoot for *at least* thirty minutes of some kind of exercise every day.

Don't supplement with iodine. Many "holistic" nutrition websites recommend that you take supplemental iodine or kelp to support your thyroid. Don't. The average American diet has plenty of iodine—and when the thyroid gland senses high levels of iodine in the blood, it will release even less thyroid hormone. Choose iodized salt instead of kosher salt to put on your food, but don't supplement to add extra.

Take other thyroid-supportive supplements. The enzyme necessary to convert T4 to T3 needs selenium to function properly. Other helpful supplements include vitamin D, zinc, and fish oil. (See the thyroid-trigger foods chart on page 146 for advice on how to get these nutrients plus other nutritional support suggestions.) As always, be sure to ask your doctor before you take any supplements, especially if you are on thyroid medication.

If you take at least 1 gram of fish oil per day, you not only help support your thyroid, you also help reduce your risk of heart attack, stroke, and other cardiovascular disease. I recommend fish oil for everyone. And when you select your multivitamin, make sure it has selenium (up to 200 micrograms) and zinc (up to 40 milligrams).

As far as your vitamin D goes, get it the old-fashioned way: Go outside each day for at least ten minutes of unprotected time in the sun. Your skin can synthesize D_3 when it is exposed to UVB rays from sunlight. You can also supplement, but be sure not to exceed the daily upper limit of 2,000 IU per day.

Combine thyroid medications. Since my diagnosis at thirty, thyroid medication has made a world of difference to me. Work with your doctor to choose the right thyroid replacement, and you may see relief in as few as two weeks. Many people benefit from a combination of both the inactive T4, found in Synthroid or Levothroid, and the active hormone T3, found in other medications such as Cytomel (100 percent T3) and Armour Thyroid (a bioidentical hormone that is 60 percent T4 and 40 percent T3). Because T3 does not show up on blood tests, it's not on some doctors' radar and they're loath to prescribe it. If your doctor objects, ask why. (And get a second opinion.)

MASTERING METABOLIC SYNDROME

We've talked a lot about insulin resistance throughout this book. Perhaps one of the most dangerous conditions that is linked to insulin resistance is metabolic syndrome (what's sometimes called syndrome X). You have metabolic syndrome when you have three or more of these risk factors:

A sizable belly. If you are an "apple," with a waist measuring more than 35 inches as a woman or 40 inches as a man, you're already in harm's way. Pile on any additional risk factors, such as smoking, being older, or of South Asian, Mexican, or Native American descent, or having diabetes in the family, and your threshold drops to 31 to 35 inches for women or to 37 or 39 inches for men.

High triglycerides. If you've already been diagnosed and treated for triglycerides, you have this risk factor, even if your level is lower than the 150 milligrams per deciliter (mg/dL) threshold.

Low HDL. If you've already been diagnosed and treated for low (good) HDL, you have this risk factor, even if your level is higher than the 50 mg/dL (as a woman) or 40 mg/dL (as a man) threshold.

High blood pressure. If you've already been diagnosed and treated for high blood pressure, you have this risk factor, even if your pressure is lower than the 130/85 threshold. (If either number is higher than the threshold—even if the other one is lower—you have this risk factor.)

High fasting blood sugar. If you've already been diagnosed and treated for high blood sugar, you have this risk factor, even if your fasting blood glucose is lower than the 100 mg/dL threshold. (If you test between 100 and 125 mg/dL, you're prediabetic; if your fasting blood test shows 126 mg/dL more than once, you're officially diabetic.)

Are you in this group? You're not alone—nearly one in four Americans has metabolic syndrome, but not many of them know it. The frightening thing about metabolic syndrome is that if you do have it, you now are twice as likely to develop heart disease and five times as likely to develop diabetes as those who do not have it. You also have a higher chance of developing fatty liver disease and PCOS. And some severe cardiovascular damage may have already been done before you even knew you had it—several studies have found that hardening of the arteries begins well before insulin resistance shows up as high fasting blood sugar. That's why it's so important to take any one of these symptoms very seriously and head off metabolic syndrome before it starts—and here are some ways to do just that.

Lose just 5 percent of your weight (preferably more!). Losing this amount of weight can reduce your risk of developing diabetes by 58 percent, reduce your risk of stroke, and reduce or completely eliminate your need for blood pressure medication. Lose 10 percent and you cut your overall risk of developing heart disease and increase your life expectancy. Shooting for that 10 percent weight loss in a year—if not sooner—is your top priority for treatment, with an ultimate goal of a BMI under 25.

Manage your insulin response. The uniting theme in all of the risk factors for metabolic syndrome is an increased risk of insulin resistance. If you follow this book's diet, especially eating smaller meals every four hours to keep your blood sugar stable, you'll lessen the amount of insulin your body needs and may radically change some of these readings very quickly. Make sure to eat some amount of protein at every meal or snack, use cinnamon, garlic, and fiber frequently, and quit smoking—all of these steps help lower blood sugar and manage insulin resistance.

Get more sleep and lower stress. Stress is linked to increased body fat, where your stomach has more receptors for cortisol. Reducing your stress level can automatically shrink your waist and lessen the amount of dangerous visceral fat, which is linked to systemic inflammation and decreased insulin sensitivity. If you pair that with a solid seven-plus hours of sleep a night, you'll lower hunger hormones cortisol and ghrelin, making it easier to stick to a healthy, low-crap diet.

Exercise! The more muscle you have, the more cells are available to absorb glucose. Exercise increases your cells' ability to use insulin, so you won't have to produce as much in response to meals. When you produce less insulin, you lower your chances of developing diabetes. (Note: If you're in the market for a step-by-step exercise program, log on to my website at www.JillianMichaels.com for a personal program that you can customize to your own level of fitness. Or check out my first two books.)

Consider extra hormonal help. Normally, I'm not a big cheerleader for drugs, but in the case of metabolic syndrome, maybe hormones can help. Recent research shows that men with metabolic syndrome and diabetes are also at risk for lower levels of testosterone. A placebo-controlled study recently found that diabetic men or those with metabolic syndrome who used a testosterone gel for fourteen days had increased insulin sensitivity—and those results lasted for a full year of treatment afterward. (Bonus: It might improve your sex life, too.) Regardless of whether you're a man or a woman, it wouldn't hurt anyone with metabolic syndrome to take advantage of the natural testosterone boost of intensive exercise and the testosterone-trigger foods on page 127.

MASTERING PCOS (POLYCYSTIC OVARIAN SYNDROME)

Polycystic ovarian syndrome is one of the most common hormonal problems in women—one in ten premenopausal women in America has it. Women may find out they have PCOS when they have trouble getting pregnant. It is the number one cause of female infertility because women with the condition don't ovulate or menstruate regularly. But girls as young as eleven have also been known to develop this condition—they typically find out when they develop severe acne or excessive facial hair.

PCOS is usually characterized by a combination of two hormonal dysfunctions—insulin resistance and androgen excess. What comes first? No one knows for sure. One theory argues that extra insulin stimulates the ovaries to produce extra testosterone. Another theory says the conditions starts in the hypothalamus. But not all women with PCOS have insulin resistance and not all of them are overweight. That's why some doctors believe that in ten years we'll have a PCOS type 1 and type 2, much like we have type 1 and type 2 diabetes now.

One thing is for sure—women who have PCOS start to experience a lot of collateral damage from their condition, in the form of these symptoms:

Abdominal obesity	Thinning hair on head	Skin tags
Acne	Higher LDL	Excessive snoring/sleep apnea
Infertility	Dandruff	Higher triglycerides
Irregular or missed periods	Oily skin	Lower HDL
Weight gain or difficulty losing weight	Excess hair on upper lip, chin, chest, back, stomach, thumbs, or toes	Darkened skin on neck, arms, breasts, or thighs

Some of these symptoms can be a hassle, but the long-term health concerns of PCOS are even worse—women with PCOS are up to seven times more likely to suffer from a heart attack than women without the condition. Pregnant women who have it face a steeper rate of miscarriage, gestational diabetes, preeclampsia, and premature delivery. More than 50 percent of women with PCOS will develop prediabetes or diabetes by the time they're forty. Managing your symptoms will not only help you feel better right now, it will reduce your likelihood of developing these serious complications.

If you suspect that you have PCOS, make an appointment with an endocrinologist and ask him or her to test your androgen and blood glucose levels for signs of insulin resistance. Other hormones that may be tested include luteinizing hormone (LH), estrogen, progesterone, and thyroid hormones. Your doctor may even order an ultrasound of your ovaries, which might show that you have a string of small cysts—hence the name of the disorder.

If you're pregnant (or want to be) and have PCOS, don't despair— your doctor can tell you about the various treatments at your disposal. PCOS is not curable, but some lifestyle and diet tips can help make the symptoms more manageable immediately and help prevent greater risks down the road. Give these a try, too:

Monitor your blood sugar. Even if you're not diagnosed with diabetes, you'll want to get very comfortable with a blood sugar monitor—it's a great way to keep tabs on how your diet influences your insulin response. Be sure to lean toward higher-protein meals and snacks—when women with PCOS used higher protein/lower carb diets to lose weight, they reduced their blood sugar, lowered levels of free androgens, and maintained a healthy HDL.

Lose that 10 percent. The Department of Health and Human Services says that even a 10 percent drop in weight can help to make your menstrual cycle more regular—not to mention improve your body's insulin sensitivity. Definitely use this book's diet, but don't forget to exercise. One study of women with PCOS found that doing just thirty minutes on a stationary bike three times a week netted them an average loss of 4.5 percent of their body weight and improved their insulin sensitivity significantly without even dieting.

Quit smoking. Think of your increased heart attack risk! Smoking jacks up your blood pressure and heart rate, raises testosterone, cortisol, and other adrenal hormones, causes insulin resistance, and messes with your ovarian function—in other words, it makes every aspect of PCOS worse. Just don't do it.

Stick to organic dairy. Insulin-like growth factor (IGF-1) stimulates the production of certain skin cells that can plug skin ducts and lead to acne. While no link has been proven between rBST hormones in dairy and PCOS, cows that are treated with growth hormones do produce milk with higher levels of IGF-1. Given the many other reasons to choose organic dairy, less acne is just icing on the cake.

► MASTERING MENOPAUSE

Muscles droop, your sex drive diminishes, and weight seems to pack on your belly, rear, and thighs no matter what you do. That's right—you're headed for menopause. Menopause naturally happens to all women between the ages of forty and fifty-five, and during the years preceding menopause—aka perimenopause—all of us face some degree of unpleasant symptoms, some more dramatically than others.

Shorter periods	Thinning hair
Longer periods	Facial hair
Heavier periods	Fuzzy thinking
Lighter periods	Moodiness
Hot flashes and night sweats	Loss of muscle tone
Insomnia	Abdominal obesity
Vaginal dryness	

Many of these symptoms, especially the night sweats and vaginal dryness, are believed to happen because our ovaries stop producing estrogen and progesterone—and, to a lesser extent, testosterone. When you've gone twelve months or more without a period, you're considered fully menopausal.

After we go through menopause, we're at greater risk for a number of conditions: breast cancer, hypothyroidism, metabolic syndrome, and diabetes. The loss of estrogen can also lead to osteoporosis and heart disease, which is why menopausal hormone therapy used to be standard care for women. That is, until 2002, when the Women's Health Initiative study found that women taking hormones faced much higher risks of heart disease, stroke, blood clots, and cancer. Now women are seeking out alternatives, and many are learning about antiaging medicine. (See "What About Bioidentical Hormones," page 44.) But why not start with some of these diet and lifestyle tips, choices that not only help you manage menopausal symptoms but also improve your overall health?

Get enough protein. Sacropenia, or loss of muscle as we age, has been seen as an inevitable outcome of aging, but a great deal of the severity is dictated by our diet and exercise. Protein helps: One study found that men and women between seventy and seventy-nine who ate the most protein lost 40 percent less lean mass than those who ate the least. Muscle burns more calories, increases your insulin sensitivity, and keeps your testosterone production higher so that you can help stave off age-related conditions such as metabolic syndrome, diabetes, and loss of libido.

Eat soy *before* menopause. Soy has phytoestrogens that may help relieve hot flashes, although studies are mixed on this issue. Stick to whole soy foods, such as tempeh and miso, and steer clear of soy bars and other products with isoflavone extracts. The active compounds in processed isoflavone products may be very different from how they are found in nature. While believed to be safe for the short term, long-term use of concentrated soy extracts has been linked to increased cancer risks, especially for women on the pill or with a family history of breast, uterine, or ovarian cancer; endometriosis; or uterine fibroids. (Ask your doctor to help you figure out if soy is okay for you.)

Don't bother with many "menopausal" supplements. Some herbs traditionally taken to relieve menopause symptoms, such as black cohosh, dong quai, and red clover, probably don't work. The National Center for Complementary and Alternative Medicine, an arm of the National Institutes of Health, looked at all the research on these three and found no evidence that they helped with hot flashes. (It also found that red clover, a phytoestrogen, carries all the same cautions as soy; black cohosh and dong quai are safe.)

One supplement that may help is ginseng, but while it may help enhance mood and sleep, it doesn't help with hot flashes. Ditto for kava, which can help lessen anxiety, but also increases your risk of liver disease. Small studies have suggested that DHEA, the precursor to estrogen and testosterone, may provide some benefit for relieving hot flashes and increasing libido, but controlled studies have shown none. Considering that it might up your risk of breast or prostate cancer, exercise caution and talk to your doctor before you start taking DHEA. The one supplement you absolutely must take is calcium with vitamin D. If you're a woman, especially if you're over thirty-five, you should be shooting for 1,200 milligrams of calcium per day. Once you hit menopause, up that to 1,500.

Use hormone creams. If you are not at risk for breast or other hormone-related cancers, but you are having trouble with hot flashes, vaginal dryness, or an overall lack of well-being, consider an estrogen cream. Applied directly to the vaginal mucous membranes, the estrogen goes where you need it most and not throughout your body, the way earlier iterations of HRT did. Many women swear by testosterone cream as well—studies have shown that it helps increase libido and relieve vaginal dryness. As with all menopausal hormone therapy, minimize any risks by asking your doctor for the smallest dosage for the shortest amount of time to be effective.

Balance energy out. The holy trinity from chapter 8—sleep, exercise, and stress relief—comes into serious play at menopause, too. Most women in this age group are caring for parents and kids at the same time. Experts say that in addition to the endorphin release you'll get, exercise also flushes out the system, and helps you manage anxiety, irritability, and depression much better.

▶ MASTERING ANDROPAUSE

Despite years of jokes and ridicule, the science is clear: Andropause, or male menopause, does exist. Unlike female menopause, which comes out of nowhere and hits women like a ton of bricks, andropause—or partial androgen deficiency, its real name—is a slow, steady decline in several key hormones.

Starting at age thirty, men's testosterone levels drop about 10 percent each decade. If a man starts to gain weight, his levels of a protein called sex hormone–binding globulin (SHBG) increase, binding with active testosterone and making it inactive. The higher the SHBG, the lower the bioavailable testosterone levels. About 30 percent of men in their fifties have noticeably lower testosterone levels, which can lead to

Decreased libido	Lagging energy
Depression	Loss of muscle mass
Erectile dysfunction	Memory loss
Insomnia	Muddy thinking

Andropause can cause changes in the testes—sperm production slows down, testicular mass shrinks, and it sometimes causes erectile dysfunction. The good news is that none of this seems to impact a guy's fertility all that much—many men go on to sire kids into their seventies. What is more likely to sideline a guy is a problem with his prostate: About 50 percent of men experience benign prostatic hypertrophy, a condition in which the prostate gets larger with scar tissue, making it more difficult to pee or ejaculate. Thyroid-stimulating hormone also declines, and cells start to lose insulin receptors, becoming less sensitive to insulin. Fasting glucose levels can rise anywhere from 6 to 14 milligrams per deciliter every ten years after age fifty. This is because the cells become less sensitive to the effects of insulin, probably due to a loss in the number of insulin receptor sites in the cell walls. Diabetes and high blood pressure—also more common among older men—can lead to erectile dysfunction, a condition few guys want. Here are a few ways to head off andropause as quickly as possible:

Exercise, would ya? Again, exercise plays a role—not only is it great for your general well-being, it also decreases your fat and helps to keep a lid on your SHBG levels so your testosterone can wander around free, not bound to any proteins. It also increases your bone and muscle strength, heading off any muscle wasting or fat building.

Don't take testosterone without a doctor's help. Doctors have seen some pretty horrific cases walking through their doors these days, after people took their testosterone supplementation into their own hands. If you're mail-ordering testosterone from, say, Bulgaria, you're essentially doping yourself with anabolic steroids. By taking steroids without a doctor's guidance, you run the risk of shutting off your own natural hormones coming from the pituitary, precursors to important chemicals you need every day.

You're effectively shutting down your own testosterone production instead of increasing it. Just say no!

Have more sex! Guys tend to have fewer erections as they get older. Up to 90 percent of erectile dysfunction comes from a physical cause, not a mental one. But doctors say being able to have decent sex when you're older is more likely if you've continued to keep your equipment in working order by having sex throughout middle age. (I know this is a hard sell, but just take one for the team, buddy.)

Eat veggie protein and fat. One study found that the best predictor of higher resting-testosterone levels was an increased level of saturated, monounsaturated, and total fat in a man's diet. Another study found that protein—but only from vegetable sources—was linked to higher levels of testosterone. (See the testosterone-trigger foods on page 127 for more suggestions on how to boost your testosterone with food.)

CHAPTER 11

WELCOME TO YOUR NEW METABOLISM

How to Carry the Remove/Restore/Rebalance Program into the Rest of Your Life

Okay, so here we are . . . at the end of the road—or should I say the beginning? Now, bolstered by the success in your diet and your lifestyle, I want you to continue these same three principles in all areas of your life. So this chapter is short and sweet. I want you to:

Remove the crap from your life—the stress, the mental and emotional clutter you carry around with you, not to mention the physical clutter that can drain all your energy.

Restore the good stuff—take the time to appreciate the life that you've just extended! You know what makes you happy—do more of it. Your hormones will automatically work a lot better.

And Rebalance—understand that even when life throws you off for a while, you have an opportunity every day to strive for that balance, to move to a middle ground where you can enjoy just enough fun and excitement to keep things interesting, but also enough rest and rejuvenation to keep yourself sane and focused.

Once you start applying these principles to your life, in all areas, you'll see that they're the only three you'll ever need—for your hormones, your health, and your happiness.

I believe in this program. I believe in you. Some of what you've read may be overwhelming, mindboggling, scary. I know. I have felt the same way. But you *do* have the power to change anything in your life that you choose to—and at any point that you choose to do so. And remember, I am right there with you fighting the good fight, walking the walk, talking the talk. Let's take back our health, reclaim our lives, shake things up, and save the world! Together we can effect change individually and globally.

You will be hot, healthy, and happy. All you have to do is be aware (which you now are) and begin incorporating these changes into your life. Some of it might be tedious, but so what? You are going to look and feel great. Isn't that worth it? And what is more important than your health? Health is the foundation your entire life rests upon. Investing in your health is committing to the pursuit of happiness. Investing in it is investing in you—what stock is more valuable?

CHAPTER 12

THE MASTER SHOPPING LIST

YOUR GRAB-AND-GO GUIDES FOR
THE FARMERS MARKET AND GROCERY STORE

Of course, your shopping list should start with the Power Nutrient food groups. I want you to buy at least some of them every time you go to the store or the farmers market. Ideally, you'll hit the farmers market first and then go to the grocery store to fill in what you couldn't find there.

To make matters totally simple, take the Master Shopping List (page 236) along—it will help you stock up on all the ingredients necessary to follow the two-week meal plan from day one. Once you're in the swing of things, you can modify it according to your tastes, as you start experimenting with new veggies and other foods.

> ## MASTER THE GROCERY STORE

Until organic farmers start getting the subsidies traditional farmers do, the only thing we can do to bring prices down is to buy more—demand goes up, supply goes up, prices go down. Here are some tips to help you get the most for your organic dollar.

Opt for store brands. Store brands of organic foods and other products are often less expensive than more well-known organic brands. Safeway's O organics line has more than three hundred products. (They're also available at Vons, Genuardi's, Dominick's, Randalls, Tom Thumb, Pavilions, and Carrs stores.) Buying these less show-offy brands not only makes good economic sense, it encourages chains to see that organic customers are price-sensitive, which will help all of us get lower prices.

Order online. If you like a certain type of food—say, beans that you know you'll eat a lot of, or brown rice—order it from an online source. You may be able to get a volume discount, and you can pick out just the varieties you like. Check out the following:

- Organic beef from www.mynaturalbeef.com
- Home delivery of organic foods in New York City from www.freshdirect.com
- Home delivery of organic foods in the Pacific Northwest from www.pioneerorganics.com
- Home delivery of organic foods in the United States and Canada from www.gobiofood.com
- Various organic offerings at www.theorganicpages.com

Haunt your local farmers market. If you go often enough and get to know the farmers at the local market, they can tell you when their specific crops are coming in. Check out www.localharvest.org.

Eat less meat. Bean-based meals can give you all of the protein at a fraction of the cost of beef, chicken, or fish. Start with one meatless meal a week, working toward one a day. You'll lessen your exposure to toxic hormones and pesticides that build up in the tissues of animal products, you'll save tons of cash, and you'll help the environment.

Make coffee at home. Don't get duped into paying five bucks for a cup of pesticide-laced coffee. Make your own organic, fair-trade coffee at home with organic whole milk or even organic half-and-half, for a luxurious but low-cost treat.

Make your own convenience foods and snacks. Single-serving containers, such as those for applesauce, cheese sticks, or yogurt, use more fossil fuels to package and ship, leach plastics into the food, and, ounce for ounce, cost more. Consider buying larger containers and serving only what you need.

The exception to the rule comes when you find yourself throwing out a lot of unused, spoiled foods. Organics don't last as long, so you have to eat them while they're fresh! If you can't eat the whole container by the time it starts to rot, stick with smaller containers or buy prewashed, presorted, precut produce, such as shredded cabbage, baby carrots, or chopped salad, that will encourage you to eat them right away.

Buy certain foods in bulk. Some stores will give you up to 5 percent off if you buy a full case or flat of a particular item. Go in on these items with friends, or even split the cost of a warehouse membership and take advantage of your own economies of scale.

Investigate food co-ops. Many areas are creating organic food co-ops. You may be able to get organic products you can't find in other stores, and because the shoppers are also the owners, prices are kept quite reasonable. (If you don't have one in your area, consider starting one. Check out the Co-operative Grocer's Information Network at www.cgin.coop/how_to_start.)

Look for a Trader Joe's. I love this store. They have really mastered the art of good-quality food at affordable prices. Many of their store brands have higher-quality ingredients at way lower prices than expensive national brands. Check out www.traderjoes.com to find the store nearest you.

Coupons? I don't know that we've hit the critical mass necessary for organic foods to warrant coupons, but I hold out hope. If you do see a coupon for an organic item, use it—doing so will only encourage other companies to offer them in the future as well. Check online at manufacturer's sites for coupons. (Stonyfield Farms has great coupons: www.stonyfield.com.) In the meantime, get a frequent-shopper's card at each of your favorite stores and use those "10 percent off your whole order" coupons, especially during weeks when you buy bulk items.

Don't buy "sticky" drinks. Juice, soda, and performance drinks all have way too much sugar that you don't need. Don't waste your money—or your resources—on bottled drinks, including water. The only beverage in a container that I'd like you to buy is organic milk. Stick with 1 percent or 2 percent organic milk, and try to find a local dairy farm, to minimize your carbon footprint and encourage the local organic economy in your area. And drink filtered water from your tap at home.

Try your hand at a veggie patch. A tomato plant might cost a couple of bucks, but you'll end up getting thirty or forty dollars' worth of home-grown tomatoes right off your back porch. Multiply that by a whole garden and you may not need to go the farmers market at all.

MASTER PROCESSED FOODS

When it comes to processed foods, very few brands pass the test for me. But with these, you know you're in good shape:

Amy's	Healthy Valley
Arrowhead Mills	Horizon
Cliff	Kashi
Eden	Luna
Erewhon	Nature's Path
Ezekiel	Newman's Own
Greens	

MEAL PLAN MASTER SHOPPING LIST

If you're ready to start the two-week meal plan, photocopy these pages to bring to the store. You have everything you need here to follow the plan to a T. (Amounts listed are for one person plus amounts for recipes; please modify according to number of people on the plan.)

SHOPPING LIST—WEEK I OF MEAL PLAN

Item (Organic Whenever Possible!)	Amount
FRESH VEGETABLES	
Asparagus	2½ pounds
Basil	1 small bunch
Carrot sticks	1 bag
Cauliflower	1 small head
Cilantro	1 small bunch

Item (Organic Whenever Possible!)	Amount
FRESH VEGETABLES	
Crimini mushrooms	2 medium
Cucumber	1 large
Eggplant	1 small
Garlic	3 heads
Green peppers	2 medium
Green beans	½ pound
Jalapeños	2 medium
Onions	3 medium
Parsley	1 small bunch
Red peppers	2 medium
Roma tomatoes	9 large
Romaine lettuce	2 heads
Salad (your choice), bagged	3 bags
Salsa, fresh	1 small container
Spinach, prewashed	2 bags
Scallions (optional)	1 bunch
Tomatoes	6 large
Zucchini	1 medium
FRESH FRUIT	
Blueberries	1½ cups
Grapefruits	1 medium
Lemons	3 medium
Oranges	2
Strawberries	1½ cups
FROZEN FOODS	
Blueberries	1 small bag
Strawberries	1 small bag
CANNED GOODS	
Albacore tuna in water	2 cans
Black beans	2 cans (15 ounces each)
Chipotle peppers in adobe sauce	1 small can
Low-sodium beef broth	1 can (14.5 ounces)
Refried black beans	1 can (15 ounces)
Tomato sauce	1 can (16 ounces)

continued on the following page

(continued)

Item (Organic Whenever Possible!)	Amount
DAIRY AND EGGS	
Eggs	2 dozen
Organic low-fat mozzarella sticks	1 package
Nonfat pepper jack cheese	1 small package (4 to 8 ounces)
Fresh Parmesan cheese (optional)	1 small piece
Plain nonfat Greek yogurt	2 containers (16 ounces each)
Reduced-fat or fat-free milk	½ gallon
MEAT/FISH	
Chicken breast	9
Chuck roast	2½ to 3 pounds
Halibut	1 serving (5 ounces)
Large prawns	10
Nitrate-free turkey bacon	1 package
Pork chop	1 5-ounce cut
Pork tenderloin	5-ounce cut
Shrimp	1 pound
Smoked turkey breast	¼ pound
Tilapia	5 ounces
Tuna fillet	5 ounces
Wild Pacific salmon	5 ounces
GRAINS/DRIED LEGUMES	
Buckwheat oats	1 package
Hummus	1 small container
Instant brown rice	1 small package
NUTS/SEEDS	
Dry roasted almonds	1 small package
Flaxseeds	1 small package
Sunflower seeds	1 small package
Walnuts	1 small package
BREAD/CEREAL/PASTA	
Ezekiel 6-inch corn tortillas	2 packages (store in fridge)
Ezekiel 7-grain bread	1 loaf (store in freezer)
Ezekiel penne pasta	1 box
Multigrain English muffins	1 package
Nature's Path flax cereal	1 box

Item (Organic Whenever Possible!)	Amount
ASSORTED OTHER ITEMS	
Applesauce	1 small jar
Balsamic vinegar	1 small bottle
Black pepper, ground	1 container
Chili powder	1 container
Cinnamon	1 container
Cornstarch	1 package
Corona Light	1 bottle
Cumin	1 container
Extra virgin olive oil	1 bottle
Honey	1 small container
Kosher salt	1 container
Lime juice	1 small bottle
Low-sodium 99 percent fat-free chicken broth	1 14.5 ounce can
Low-sodium beef broth	1 14.5 ounce can
Mint	1 bunch
Non-reduced-sodium chicken broth	1 14.5 ounce can
Nonstick cooking spray	1 bottle
Red pepper chile flakes	1 container
White vinegar	1 small bottle
Whole-grain mustard	1 small jar
Xylitol (natural sweetener)	1 container

SHOPPING LIST—WEEK 2 OF MEAL PLAN

Item (Organic Whenever Possible!)	Amount
FRESH VEGETABLES	
Artichokes	8 medium-large
Asparagus	⅔ pound
Broccoli	1 bunch
Brussels sprouts	1 small container
Carrots	1 pound
Celery	3 large stalks
Cilantro	1 bunch
Garlic	2 heads
Green beans	1 pound

continued on the following page

Item (Organic Whenever Possible!)	Amount
Green peppers	2 medium
Jalapeños	3 large
Mixed baby greens	1 bag
Onions	5 medium
Parsley (optional)	1 bunch
Poblano chile (optional)	1 small
Red peppers	2 medium
Roma tomatoes	1 medium-large
Romaine lettuce	2 large heads
Salsa, fresh	1 small container
Serrano chile	1 medium
Shallots	1 small bunch
Sun-dried tomatoes	¼ cup
Tomatoes	3 large
FRESH FRUIT	
Apples	1
Berries (your choice)	1 pint
Blueberries	1 cup
Lemons	2 medium
Limes	3 medium
Oranges	2 medium
Peaches	1
Strawberries	1 cup
Watermelon	1 small
CANNED GOODS	
Amy's Organic Medium Chili with Vegetables	1 can (15 ounces)
Amy's Organic Split Pea Soup	1 can (15 ounces)
Diced tomatoes	1 15-ounce can
Refried black beans	1 can (15 ounces)
DAIRY AND EGGS	
Low-fat organic Cheddar	1 small package (8 ounces)
Eggs	2 dozen
Nonfat plain Greek yogurt	1 container (16 ounces)
Reduced-fat or fat-free milk	½ gallon
Unsalted butter	1 stick

Item (Organic Whenever Possible!)	Amount
MEAT/FISH	
Chicken breasts	5
Flank steak	5 ounces
Grass-fed lean sirloin	1½ pounds, ground
Halibut	4 4- to 6-ounce fillets
Lean, low-sodium turkey sausage	1 small package
Prawns	5 large
Sliced turkey breast	1 pound
Tuna steak	5 ounces
Pacific wild salmon	5 ounce fillet or steak
GRAINS/DRIED LEGUMES	
Quaker instant oatmeal	8 packets
Quinoa	1 cup
NUTS/SEEDS	
Pecans	¼ cup
Raw almonds	1 small bag
BREAD/CEREAL/PASTA	
Ezekiel 8-inch corn tortillas	2 packages
ASSORTED OTHER ITEMS	
Almond butter	1 small container
Ancho chile powder	1 container
Dijon mustard	1 small jar
Galeos Ceasar Salad Dressing	1 bottle
Guiltless Gourmet baked tortilla chips	1 bag
Kashi vegetable crackers	1 box
Lemon juice	1 small bottle
Low-sodium chicken broth	1 container (8 ounces; can or pouch)
Rice wine vinegar	1 small bottle

RESOURCES

I firmly believe that in a short time, everybody will come around to the organic, natural way of eating. Given the evidence, how can they not? In the meantime, it might be a bit tricky to find the food you need where you live. Not to mention the personal- and home-care products that don't have all those endocrine-disrupting chemicals. I've compiled a short list of good places to go to get information, products, and other resources to help you lead the way.

ORGANIC AND SUSTAINABLE FOOD AND PRODUCTS

www.nrdc.org/health/foodmiles
The National Resources Defense Council has developed a minisite to help you find organic foods in your area. You can look up your state and the time of year to find out what foods are in season locally.

www.earthlab.com
Calculate your carbon footprint and find tons of interesting ways to reduce it by 15 percent this year. I partner with these guys because I think they do great work.

www.panna.org
www.pesticideinfo.org
Pesticide Action Network is at the forefront of the organic food move-
ment and helps you find out how you can minimize your exposure to
highly hazardous pesticides.

www.ewg.org
www.ewg.org/sites/tapwater
(The National Tap Water Quality Database)
These guys are so bad-ass. The Environmental Working Group is at the
forefront of many amazing initiatives to inform the public about just how
bad greedy corporations are screwing the environment and our health.
(These guys were the ones who did the big study that helped teach consumers about "The Dirty Dozen," the most pesticide-laden fruits and vegetables, for example.) They recently developed a lobbying arm that's
definitely on *our* side of the toxic equation. Keep an eye out for them in
the media—they are everywhere, and they are definitely the good guys.

www.ourstolenfuture.org
This site takes its name from the book *Our Stolen Future,* an extremely
influential analysis of endocrine disruption that was first published in
1996. Since its publication, the authors (two environmental scientists
and an award-winning investigative journalist) have continued to collect
damning research about endocrine disruptors in the environment. This
site will make your hair turn white. Seriously, take a look—you'll understand much better why I'm so passionate about this topic.

www.theorganicpages.com
The Organic Trade Association (OTA) created the Organic Pages Online
to make it easier for you to find certified organic products, producers, ingredients, supplies, and services in your area. It's expanding constantly—
take a look.

www.eatlocalamerica.coop
Eat Local America is a challenge set up by the National Cooperative
Grocers Association (NCGA) to help boost local food co-op participation by asking people to consume 80 percent of their diets (or 4 out of
every 5 meals) from local foods during the summer months. Fun! Check
out their interactive map, or visit the NCGA Web site for more resources: www.ncga.coop.

www.slowfoodusa.org
www.slowfood.com
Slow Food is a group dedicated to helping people reconnect with their food. They advocate food produced in environmentally sustainable, clean practices that protect animal welfare and people's health. You'll find lots of great resources about how to make fresh, whole, locally and sustainably grown food a mainstay of your diet.

www.eatwild.com
This site has a tremendous amount of info about grass-fed beef, lamb, goats, bison, poultry, pork, dairy, and other similar foods. You'll also find tons of links to local suppliers of all-natural, grass-fed products.

www.psr.org
Physicians for Social Responsibility started with a mission of ridding the world of nuclear dangers. They've expanded to include all environmental degradation as well. These guys are lobbying government on our side— check out their site and do what you can to support them.

www.organicvalley.com
This is a favorite site of Chef Stuart O'Keeffe, an organic chef whom I work with quite often. This company is one of his favorite organic food producers, and the site contains lots of great information regarding reasons to buy organic.

www.wellnessgrocer.com
This is an online grocer devoted to organic foods and natural personal-care products.

www.foodandwaterwatch.org
Another watchdog/lobbying group that helps protect our food and water. This site has tons of helpful fact sheets, information, and reports on food and water safety.

www.sustainabletable.org
www.eatwellguide.org
These sites have recipes, shopping guides, maps to hormone-free dairies, farmers markets, food co-ops, and tons of other stuff. The Eat Well Guide is a free online directory of sustainably raised meat, poultry,

dairy, and eggs from farms, stores, restaurants, bed-and-breakfasts, and more in the United States and Canada. Just enter your zip or postal code to find healthy products in your town or wherever you're going to be traveling to.

www.checnet.org/healtheHouse/pdf/plasticchart.pdf
This fantastic chart spells out the best and worst plastic products on the market for home use.

www.truefoodnow.org/genetically-engineered-foods/shoppers-guide/
This site provides an extremely helpful, huge list of nongenetically engineered foods.

www.organic-center.org
This site is an incredible trove of interesting resources about organics. The organization is funded by many natural-food producers in an effort to further knowledge of organic agricultural methods.

www.organicconsumers.org
Buyer's guides for everything from food to clothing to cleaning products. You will find Community Supported Agriculture (CSAs), organic home delivery, building materials, and resources. The Organic Consumers Association and GreenPeople.org have compiled one of the world's largest directories of green and organic businesses.

www.newdream.org
This amazing organization has been working to try to convince Americans to live simply for more than a decade. They provide many great resources and really smart, creative thinking to individuals, institutions, communities, and businesses about how to "consume responsibly to protect the environment, enhance quality of life, and promote social justice." (They even have a wallet card you can print out with this smart personal credo: "Every dollar I spend is a statement about the kind of world I want and the quality of life I value.")

apps.ams.usda.gov/FarmersMarkets
This is a great searchable database of farmers markets throughout the United States that's maintained and updated regularly by the government.

www.organicexchange.org
This is a great resource for those interested in organic cotton, including buyer's guides for organic cotton clothing.

www.localharvest.org
This site has a clickable interactive map that helps you locate your nearest farmers market. They also have a ton of info about CSAs, family farms, and other sources of sustainably grown food in your area.

▶ NONTOXIC-PRODUCT RESOURCES

www.amazon.com/tag/bpa-free/products
Amazon.com has compiled a list of hundreds of BPA-free products for one-stop shopping.

www.healthychild.org
The Healthy Child, Healthy World program offers information and resources for parents who want to create a healthy, nontoxic environment for their kids—and for themselves, too.

www.householdproducts.nlm.nih.gov
This government site has a complete database of household products with safety and handling suggestions.

▶ OTHER HELPFUL RESOURCES

www.calorieking.com
I recommend this site (as well as the companion book, *The Calorie King Calorie, Fat & Carbohydrate Counter* by Allan Borushek) to everyone on *Biggest Loser.* You can find great nutrient information about thousands of foods. Use the site at home; buy the book for when you're out on the town. Even if you're not watching calories, having a general gauge of nutrients is very useful.

PERSONAL PROGRAM

www.JillianMichaels.com
You can get tons of up-to-date information, tools, and trackers, and customized meal plans on my site. You can even add a personal coach, if you'd like!

SELECTED REFERENCES

CHAPTER I

Alexander, D., Manier, J., and Callahan, P. "For Every Fad, Another Cookie: How Science and Diet Crazes Confuse Consumers, Reshape Recipes and Fail, Ultimately, to Reform Eating Habits." *Chicago Tribune,* August 23, 2005.

American Institute for Cancer Research. "A Closer Look at Nutrigenomics: How Nutrients and Genes Interact." 2008. www.aicr.org/site/PageServer?pagename= pub_A_Closer_Look_At_Nutrigenomics.

Berkowitz, R. "Growth of Children at High Risk of Obesity during the First 6 Years of Life: Implications for Prevention." *American Journal of Clinical Nutrition* 81, no. 1 (January 2005).

BJC Behavioral Health. "Calorie Needs: Calculate Your Basal Metabolic Rate." BJC HealthCare. http://www.bjcbehavioralhealth.org/behavioralhealth_wellness.aspx ?id=1993/.

Bouchez, C. "Make the Most of Your Metabolism." WebMD. www.webmd.com/ fitness-exercise/guide/make-most-your-metabolism/ (February 24, 2006).

Canaris, G., et al. "The Colorado Thyroid Disease Prevalence Study." *Archives of Internal Medicine* 160, no. 4 (February 28, 2000).

Carroll, J. "How Many Different Times, If Any, Have You Seriously Tried to Lose Weight in Your Life?" (self-reported lifetime number of weight-loss attempts, 1990, 1999, and 2005). The Gallup Organization, August 16, 2005.

Centers for Disease Control. "Prevalence of Overweight Among Children and Adolescents: United States, 2003–2004." www.cdc.gov/nchs/products/pubs/pubd/ hestats/overweight/overwght_child_03.htm.

Chandola, T., Brunner, E., and Marmot, M. "Chronic Stress at Work and the Metabolic Syndrome: Prospective Study." *British Medical Journal* 332 (March 4, 2006).

Delinsky, S., Latner, J., and Wilson, G. "Binge Eating and Weight Loss in a Self-Help Behavior Modification Program." *Obesity* 14, no. 7 (July 2006).

DeNoon, D. "Diet Soda Drinkers Gain Weight, Overweight Risk Soars 41 Percent with Each Daily Can of Diet Soda." CBSNews.com, June 13, 2005. www.cbsnews.com/stories/2005/06/13/health/webmd/main701408.shtml.

Fantuzzi, G., and Faggioni, R. "Leptin in the Regulation of Immunity, Inflammation, and Hematopoiesis." *Journal of Leukocyte Biology* 68, no. 4 (October 2000).

Farah, H., and Buzby, J. "U.S. Food Consumption Up 16 Percent since 1970." Amber Waves (USDA Economic Research Service), November 2005.

Ferrini, R., and Barrett-Connor, E. "Sex Hormones and Age: A Cross-Sectional Study of Testosterone and Estradiol and Their Bioavailable Fractions in Community-Dwelling Men." *American Journal of Epidemiology* 147, no. 8 (April 15, 1998).

Fox, M., et al. "Feeding Infants and Toddlers Study: What Foods Are Infants and Toddlers Eating?" Suppl. 1, *Journal of the American Dietetic Association* 104, no. 1 (January 2004).

Gable, S., Chang, Y., and Krull, J. "Television Watching and Frequency of Family Meals Are Predictive of Overweight Onset and Persistence in a National Sample of School-Aged Children." *Journal of the American Dietetic Association* 107, no. 1 (January 2007).

Gluckman, P., et al. "Metabolic Plasticity during Mammalian Development Is Directionally Dependent on Early Nutritional Status." *Proceedings of the National Academy of Sciences USA* 104, no. 31 (July 31, 2007).

Goulden, V., Layton, A., Cunliffe, W. "Long-Term Safety of Isotretinoin as a Treatment for Acne Vulgaris." *British Journal of Dermatology* 131, no. 3 (September 1994).

Hall Moran, V., Leathard, H., and Coley, J. "Urinary Hormone Levels during the Natural Menstrual Cycle: The Effect of Age." *Journal of Endocrinology* 170, no. 1 (July 2001).

Henig, R. "Fat Factors." *New York Times*, August 13, 2006.

Hofferth, S., and Curtin, S. "Sports Participation and Child Overweight: 1997–2002." www.authorstream.com/Presentation/Saverio-45025-Network-meeting-sept152005-Child-sports-participat-Participation-Overweight-1997-2002-Objectives-Education-ppt-powerpoint.

Isaacs, S. *Hormonal Balance*. Boulder, CO: Bull Publishing Company, 2007.

Kaiser Family Foundation. "The Role of Media in Childhood Obesity" (issue brief, February 2004). www.kff.org/entmedia/upload/The-Role-Of-Media-in-Childhood-Obesity.pdf.

Kant, A. "Reported Consumption of Low-Nutrient-Density Foods by American Children and Adolescents: Nutritional and Health Correlates, NHANES III, 1988 to 1994." *Archives of Pediatrics and Adolescent Medicine* 157, no. 8 (August 2003).

Karras, T. "The Disorder Next Door." *Self,* May 2008.

Kubik, M., Lytle, L., and Story, M. "Schoolwide Food Practices Are Associated with Body Mass Index in Middle School Students." *Archives of Pediatric Adolescent Medicine* 159, no. 12 (2005).

Lallukka, T., et al. "Psychosocial Working Conditions and Weight Gain among Employees." *International Journal of Obesity* 29, no. 8 (August 2005).

Lumeng, J., et al. "Association between Clinically Meaningful Behavior Problems and Overweight in Children." *Pediatrics* 112, no. 5 (November 2003).

Lutgen-Sandvik, P., Tracy, S., and Alberts, J. "Burned by Bullying in the American Workplace: Prevalence, Perception, Degree, and Impact." *Journal of Management Studies* 44, no. 6 (September 2007).

Macleod, M. "Why Are Girls Growing Up So Fast?" *New Scientist,* February 10, 2007.

Manier, J., Callahan, P., and Alexander, D. "The Oreo, Obesity and Us: Craving the

Cookie: The Brain Is Wired to Love Sweets, but Are They Addictive? America's Iconic Cookie Captures the Nation's Burgeoning Dietary Dilemma." *Chicago Tribune,* August 21, 2005.

Ogden, C., Carroll, M., and Flegal, K. "High Body Mass Index for Age Among US Children and Adolescents, 2003–2006." *Journal of the American Medical Association* 299, no. 20 (2008).

Peterson, M., et al. "Our Stolen Future: A Decade Later." *San Francisco Medicine* (in press).

Prasad, A., et al. "Zinc Status and Serum Testosterone Levels of Healthy Adults." *Nutrition* 12, no. 5 (May 1996).

Reed, D., Lawler, M., and Tordoff, M. "Reduced Body Weight Is a Common Effect of Gene Knockout in Mice." *BMC Genetics* 9 (January 8, 2008).

Ribeiro, L., et al. "Impact of Acute Exercise Intensity on Plasma Concentrations of Insulin, Growth Hormone and Somatostatin," *Acta Médica Portuguesa* 17, no. 3 (May–June 2004).

Roizen, M., and Oz, M. *You: On a Diet: The Owner's Manual for Waist Management.* New York: Free Press, 2006.

Snoek, H. "Parental Behaviour and Adolescents' Emotional Eating." *Appetite* 49, no. 1 (July 2007).

Spalding, K., et al. "Dynamics of Fat Cell Turnover in Humans." *Nature* 453, no. 7196 (June 5, 2008).

Tabarrok, A. "A Brief Report on Economic Research on Obesity." The Independent Institute, March 31, 2003. www.independent.org/newsroom/article.asp?id=1153.

Taubes, G. "What If It's All Been a Big Fat Lie?" *New York Times,* July 7, 2002.

The Obesity Society. "Obesity, Society, and Stigmatization." www.obesity.org/information/weight_bias.asp.

University of Maryland Medical Center Patient Education. "Diabetes Type 2." University of Maryland Medical Center. www.umm.edu/patiented/articles/what_causes_type_2_diabetes_000060_2.htm (July 15, 2006).

CHAPTER 2

Associated Press. "Appetite-Suppressing Hormone Discovered." www.msnbc.msn.com/id/9993771 (November 10, 2005).

Associated Press. "Irregular Sleep Tied to Obesity, Other Health Problems." *USA Today,* May 7, 2008. www.usatoday.com/news/health/2008-05-07-sleep-obesity_N.htm.

Bell, G., et al. "End-Organ Responses to Thyroxine Therapy in Subclinical Hypothyroidism." *Clinical Endocrinology* 22, no. 1 (January 1985).

Biddinger, S., et al. "Hepatic Insulin Resistance Is Sufficient to Produce Dyslipidemia and Susceptibility to Atherosclerosis." *Cell Metabolism* 7, no. 2 (February 2008).

Burstain, T. "Balancing Your Hunger Hormones." www.hungerhormones.com (accessed Nov. 21, 2008).

Center for Bioenvironmental Research, Tulane and Xavier Universities. "E.hormone: your gateway to the environment and your hormones." www.e.hormone.tulane.edu (accessed Nov. 21, 2008).

Conrad, C. "Overture for Growth Hormone: Requiem for Interleukin-6?" *Critical Care Medicine* 35, no. 12 (December 2007).

Davis, C., and Saltos, E. "Dietary Recommendations and How They Have Changed over Time." USDA Economic Research Service. http://www.ers.usda.gov/publications/AIB750/AIB750B.PDF (May 1999).

Doucet, E., and Cameron, J. "Appetite Control after Weight Loss: What Is the Role of Bloodborne Peptides?" *Applied Physiology, Nutrition, and Metabolism* 32, no. 3 (June 2007).

Enriori, P., et al. "Diet-Induced Obesity Causes Severe but Reversible Leptin Resistance in Arcuate Melanocortin Neurons." *Cell Metabolism* 5, no. 3 (March 2007).

Environmental Working Group. "What's the Difference?" www.foodnews.org.

ESHRE Capri Workshop Group. "Nutrition and Reproduction in Women." *Human Reproduction Update* 12, no. 3 (May–June 2006).

"Estrogen." www.labtestsonline.org.

Feldman, H. "Age Trends in the Level of Serum Testosterone and Other Hormones in Middle-Aged Men: Longitudinal Results from the Massachusetts Male Aging Study." *Journal of Clinical Endocrinology and Metabolism* 87 (2) (February 2002).

Foster, G. "A Policy-Based School Intervention to Prevent Overweight and Obesity." *Pediatrics* 121 (April 2008): e794–e802.

Grady, D. "In Study, Hormone Reduced Appetite in Mice." *New York Times,* November 11, 2005.

Henry, J. "Biological Basis of the Stress Response: Address upon Accepting the Hans Selye Award from the American Institute of Stress in Montreux, Switzerland, February 1991." *Integrative Psychological and Behavioral Science* 27, no. 1 (January 1992).

Isaacs, S. *The Leptin Boost Diet.* Berkeley, CA: Ulysses Press, 2007.

LoCicero, K. "The Role of Hormones in Weight Management." *NutriNews: Recent Health and Nutrition Information from Douglas Laboratories,* March 2007.

Lutter, M., et al. "The Orexigenic Hormone Ghrelin Defends against Depressive Symptoms of Chronic Stress." *Nature Neuroscience* 11, no. 7 (July 2008).

Matsuzawa, Y., et al. "Adiponectin and Metabolic Syndrome." *Arteriosclerosis, Thrombosis, and Vascular Biology* 24, no. 1 (January 2004).

Mayo Clinic Health Letter, June 2008.

Mayo Clinic staff. "DHEA." MayoClinic.com. www.mayoclinic.com/health/dhea/NS_patient-dhea401 (January 1, 2008).

Mirsky, S. "Vicious Circle of Belly Fat." *Scientific American,* April 17, 2008.

National Digestive Diseases Information Clearinghouse (NDDIC). "Your Digestive System and How It Works." NIH publication no. 08–2681, April 2008. digestive.niddk.nih.gov/ddiseases/pubs/yrdd/.

Nussey, S., and Whitehead, S. "Hypothalamic Control of Adrenocortical Steroid Synthesis—CRH and Vasopressin." *Endocrinology: An Integrated Approach.* Oxford, UK: BIOS Scientific Publishers Ltd, 2001. www.ncbi.nlm.nih.gov/books/bv.fcgi?rid=endocrin.section.516 (accessed November 21, 2008).

Overduin, J., et al. "Role of the Duodenum and Macronutrient Type in Ghrelin Regulation." *Endocrinology* 146, no. 2 (February 2005).

Physicians for Social Responsibility. "Environmental Endocrine Disruptors: What Health Care Providers Should Know." www.psr.org/site/DocServer/Environmental_Endocrine_Disruptors.pdf.

Roizen, M., and Oz, M. *You: On a Diet: The Owner's Manual for Waist Management.* New York: Free Press, 2006.

Romero-Corral, A., et al. "Normal Weight Obesity: A Risk Factor for Cardiometabolic Dysregulations." American College of Cardiology Annual Scientific Session, Chicago, IL, April 1, 2008.

Rönnemaa, E., et al. "Impaired Insulin Secretion Increases the Risk of Alzheimer Disease." *Neurology,* April 9, 2008.

Saudek, C. D., et al. "A New Look at Screening and Diagnosing Diabetes Mellitus." *Journal of Clinical Endocrinology and Metabolism* (May 6, 2008).

Spiegel, K., et al. "Brief Communication: Sleep Curtailment in Healthy Young Men Is Associated with Decreased Leptin Levels, Elevated Ghrelin Levels, and Increased Hunger and Appetite." *Annals of Internal Medicine* 141, no. 11 (December 7, 2004).

The Merck Manual of Medical Information. http://www.merck.com/mmhe/index.html.

Tran, T., et al. "Beneficial Effects of Subcutaneous Fat Transplantation on Metabolism." *Cell Metabolism* 7, no. 5 (May 2008).

Tschop, M., et al. "Diet-Induced Leptin Resistance: The Heart of the Matter." *Endocrinology* 148, no. 3 (March 2007).

Weight Control Information Network. "New Hormone Provides Clues About Weight Loss." *WIN Notes* (winter 2002–2003). win.niddk.nih.gov/notes/winter03notes/newhormone.htm.

Westling, B., et al. "Low CSF Leptin in Female Suicide Attempters with Major Depression." *Journal of Affective Disorders* 81, no. 1 (July 2004).

CHAPTER 3

Alexander, D., Manier, J., and Callahan, P. "For Every Fad, Another Cookie: How Science and Diet Crazes Confuse Consumers, Reshape Recipes and Fail, Ultimately, to Reform Eating Habits." *Chicago Tribune,* August 23, 2005.

Alonso-Magdalena, P., et al. "The Estrogenic Effect of Bisphenol-A Disrupts the Pancreatic ß-Cell Function *In Vivo* and Induces Insulin Resistance." *Environmental Health Perspectives* 114 (2006).

American Physiological Society. "Treatment with an Antipsychotic Drug Found to Cause Changes in Metabolism Earlier Than Expected." American Physiological Society. www.the-aps.org/press/journal/08/15.htm (April 7, 2008).

Amorim, A., et al. "Does Excess Pregnancy Weight Gain Constitute a Major Risk for Increasing Long-Term BMI?" *Obesity* 15 (2007) (May 2007).

Bauer, S. (ed.) *National Geographic Green Guide.* www.thegreenguide.com.

Berkowitz, R. "Growth of Children at High Risk of Obesity during the First 6 Years of Life: Implications for Prevention." *American Journal of Clinical Nutrition* 81, no. 1 (January 2005).

Brunner, E., et al. "Prospective Effect of Job Strain on General and Central Obesity in the Whitehall II Study." *American Journal of Epidemiology* 165, no. 7 (April 1, 2007).

Bulayeva, N., and Watson, C. "Xenoestrogen-Induced ERK-1 and ERK-2 Activation via Multiple Membrane-Initiated Signaling Pathways." *Environmental Health Perspectives* 112, no. 15 (November 2004).

Callahan, P., Manier, J., and Alexander, D. "Where There's Smoke, There Might Be Food Research, Too: Documents Indicate Kraft, Philip Morris Shared Expertise on How the Brain Processes Tastes, Smells." *Chicago Tribune,* January 29, 2006.

Center for Bioenvironmental Research, Tulane and Xavier Universities. "E.hormone: Your Gateway to the Environment and Your Hormones." www.e.hormone.tulane.edu.

Centers for Disease Control. "Prevalence of Overweight Among Children and Adolescents: United States, 2003–2004." www.cdc.gov/nchs/products/pubs/pubd/hestats/overweight/overwght_child_03.htm.

Centers for Disease Control. "Third National Report on Human Exposure to Environmental Chemicals: Spotlight on Organochlorine Pesticides." July 2005. www. cdc.gov/ExposureReport/pdf/factsheet_organochlorine.pdf.

Chamie, K., deVere White, R., and Ellison, L. "Agent Orange Exposure, Vietnam War Veterans and the Risk of Prostate Cancer." Abstract 421, suppl., *Journal of Urology* 179 (2008).

Chaput, J. "The Association Between Sleep Duration and Weight Gain in Adults: A 6-Year Prospective Study from the Quebec Family Study." *Sleep* 31 (4): 517–23 (April 11, 2008).

Chen, J. "Maternal Burden of Organochloro-Compounds Associated with Unde-scended Testes." Abstract 276, suppl., *Journal of Urology* 179 (2008).

Chiolero, A. "Consequences of Smoking for Body Weight, Body Fat Distribution, and Insulin Resistance." *American Journal of Clinical Nutrition* 87, no. 4 (April 2008).

DeCaro, J., et al. "Maternal Exposure to Polybrominated Biphenyls and Genitourinary Conditions in Male Offspring." Abstract 277, suppl., *Journal of Urology* 179 (2008).

Dewey, K. "Is Breastfeeding Protective against Child Obesity?" *Journal of Human Lactation* 19, no. 1 (February 2003).

Donn, J., Mendoza, M., and Pritchard, J. "Drugs Found in Drinking Water." *USA Today,* March 10, 2008.

Environment California Research and Policy Center. "Bisphenol-A Overview." www. environmentcalifornia.org.

Environmental Working Group. "A Survey of Bisphenol A in U.S. Canned Foods." March 5, 2007. www.ewg.org/reports/bisphenola.

Feldman, H. "Age Trends in the Level of Serum Testosterone and Other Hormones in Middle-Aged Men: Longitudinal Results from the Massachusetts Male Aging Study." *Journal of Clinical Endocrinology and Metabolism* 87 (2) (February 2002).

Field, A., et al. "Association of Weight Change, Weight Control Practices, and Weight Cycling among Women in the Nurses' Health Study II." *International Journal of Obesity and Related Metabolic Disorders* 28, no. 9 (September 2004).

Flier, J., and Elmquist, J. "A Good Night's Sleep: Future Antidote to the Obesity Epi-demic?" *Annals of Internal Medicine* 141, no. 11 (December 7, 2004).

Heilbronn, L., et al. "Effect of 6-Month Calorie Restriction on Biomarkers of Longevity, Metabolic Adaptation, and Oxidative Stress in Overweight Individu-als." *Journal of the American Medical Association* 295, no. 13 (April 5, 2006).

Henig, R. "Fat Factors." *New York Times,* August 13, 2006.

Hoponick, J. "Nonylphenol Ethoxylates: A Safer Alternative Exists to This Toxic Clean-ing Agent." Sierra Club, November 2005. www.sierraclub.org/toxics/nonylphenol_ethoxylates3.pdf.

International Food Information Council. "2008 Food & Health Survey: Consumer At-titudes toward Food, Nutrition, and Health." May 14, 2008. http://www.ific.org.

International Obesity TaskForce. "Endocrine Disruptors in Common Plastics Linked to Obesity Risk." *ScienceDaily,* May 15, 2008, and May 22, 2008. www. sciencedaily.com/releases/2008/05/080514091427.htm.

Isaacs, S. *Hormonal Balance.* Boulder, CO: Bull Publishing Company, 2007.

Isaacs, S. *The Leptin Boost Diet.* Berkeley, CA: Ulysses Press, 2007.

Jeffery, R., and Harnack, L. "Evidence Implicating Eating as a Primary Driver for the Obesity Epidemic." *Diabetes* 56, no. 11 (November 2007).

Kapoor, D., and Jones, T. "Smoking and Hormones in Health and Endocrine Disor-ders." *European Journal of Endocrinology* 152, no. 4 (2005).

Keith, S. "Putative Contributors to the Secular Increase in Obesity: Exploring the Roads Less Traveled." *International Journal of Obesity* 30, no. 11 (November 2006).

Khamsi, R. "Common Genetic Change Linked to Obesity." NewScientist.com news service, April 13, 2006. www.newscientist.com.

Knowler, W., et al. "Reduction in the Incidence of Type 2 Diabetes with Lifestyle Intervention or Metformin." *New England Journal of Medicine* 346, no. 6 (February 7, 2002).

Lang, S., et al. "Association of Urinary Bisphenol A Concentration with Medical Disorders and Laboratory Abnormalities in Adults." *JAMA* 300, no. 11 (September 17, 2008).

Layton, L., and Lee, C. "Canada Bans BPA from Baby Bottles." *Washington Post,* April 19, 2008.

Lee, D., et al. "Association between Serum Concentrations of Persistent Organic Pollutants and Insulin Resistance among Nondiabetic Adults: Results from the National Health and Nutrition Examination Survey 1999–2002." *Diabetes Care* 30, no. 3 (March 2007).

Lee, D., et al. "Relationship between Serum Concentrations of Persistent Organic Pollutants and the Prevalence of Metabolic Syndrome among Non-diabetic Adults: Results from the National Health and Nutrition Examination Survey 1999–2002." *Diabetologia* 50, no. 9 (September 2007).

Ley, R. "Human Gut Microbes Associated with Obesity." *Nature* 444 (7122) (December 21, 2006).

Mably, T., et al. "In Utero and Lactational Exposure of Male Rats to 2,3,7, 8-Tetrachlorodibenzo-p-dioxin. 3. Effects on Spermatogenesis and Reproductive Capability." *Toxicology and Applied Pharmacology* 114, no. 1 (May 1992).

Manier, J., Callahan, P., and Alexander, D. "The Oreo, Obesity and Us: Craving the Cookie: The Brain Is Wired to Love Sweets, but Are They Addictive? America's Iconic Cookie Captures the Nation's Burgeoning Dietary Dilemma." *Chicago Tribune,* August 21, 2005.

Martin, F-P., et al. "Probiotic Modulation of Symbiotic Gut Microbial-Host Metabolic Interactions in a Humanized Microbiome Mouse Model." *Molecular Systems Biology* 4 (2008).

Mayo Clinic staff. "Lose a Little; Helps a Lot." *Mayo Clinic Health Letter,* January 2008.

McDougall, G., and Stewart, D. "The Inhibitory Effects of Berry Polyphenols on Digestive Enzymes." *Biofactors* 23, no. 4 (2005).

Mendola, P., et al. "Consumption of PCB-Contaminated Freshwater Fish and Shortened Menstrual Cycle Length." *American Journal of Epidemiology* 146, no. 11 (December 1, 1997).

Montgomery, M., et al. "Incident Diabetes and Pesticide Exposure among Licensed Pesticide Applicators: Agricultural Health Study, 1993–2003." *American Journal of Epidemiology* 167, no. 10 (May 15, 2008).

Neumark-Sztainer, D., et al. "Accurate Parental Classification of Overweight Adolescents' Weight Status: Does It Matter?" *Pediatrics* 121, no. 6 (June 2008).

Ozelli, K. "This Is Your Brain on Food: Neuroimaging Reveals Shared Basis for Chocoholia and Drug Addiction." *Scientific American,* August 19, 2007.

Pasarica, M., and Dhurandhar, N. "Infectobesity: Obesity of Infectious Origin." *Advances in Food and Nutrition Research* 52 (2007).

Pesticide Action Network North America. "Case Study: Organochlorine Pesticides." www.chemicalbodyburden.org/cs_organochl.htm.

Physicians for Social Responsibility. "Environmental Endocrine Disruptors: What Health Care Providers Should Know." www.psr.org/site/DocServer/Environmental_ Endocrine_Disruptors.pdf.

Pimentel, D. "Environmental, Energetic, and Economic Comparisons of Organic and Conventional Farming Systems." *BioScience* 55, no. 7 (July 2005).

Raeder, M. "Obesity, Dyslipidemia, and Diabetes with Selective Serotonin Reuptake Inhibitors: The Hordaland Health Study." *Journal of Clinical Psychiatry* 67, no. 12 (December 2006).

Raloff, J. "Hormones: Here's the Beef: Environmental Concerns Reemerge over Steroids Given to Livestock." *Science News* 161, no. 1 (January 5, 2002).

Reuters. " 'Do More, Talk Less' to Help Heavy Teens: Parents Who Push Kids to Diet Should Instead Urge Them to Get Moving." MSNBC.com, June 4, 2008. www.msnbc.msn.com/id/24970815/.

Roizen, M., and Oz, M. *You: On a Diet: The Owner's Manual for Waist Management.* New York: Free Press, 2006.

Setlur, S., et al. "Estrogen-Dependent Signaling in a Molecularly Distinct Subclass of Aggressive Prostate Cancer." *Journal of the National Cancer Institute* 100, no. 11 (June 4, 2008).

Soto, A. "Androgenic and Estrogenic Activity in Water Bodies Receiving Cattle Feedlot Effluent in Eastern Nebraska, USA." *Environmental Health Perspectives* 112, no. 3 (March 2004).

Spiegel, K., et al. "Brief Communication: Sleep Curtailment in Healthy Young Men Is Associated with Decreased Leptin Levels, Elevated Ghrelin Levels, and Increased Hunger and Appetite." *Annals of Internal Medicine* 141, no. 11 (December 7, 2004).

Steinman, G. "Mechanisms of Twinning: VII. Effect of Diet and Heredity on the Human Twinning Rate." *Journal of Reproductive Medicine* 51, no. 5 (May 2006).

Steinman, G. "Mechanisms of Twinning: VIII. Maternal Height, Insulinlike Growth Factor and Twinning Rate." *Journal of Reproductive Medicine* 51, no. 9 (September 2006).

"Surprising Advice for Insomniacs: Sleep Less." *Harvard HealthBeat,* May 8, 2008.

Sustainable Table. "Artificial Hormones." www.sustainabletable.org/issues/hormones/index_pf.html.

Teff, K., et al. "Dietary Fructose Reduces Circulating Insulin and Leptin, Attenuates Postprandial Suppression of Ghrelin, and Increases Triglycerides in Women." *Journal of Clinical Endocrinology and Metabolism* 89, no. 6 (June 2004).

Tsai, C. "Weight Cycling and Risk of Gallstone Disease in Men." *Archives of Internal Medicine* 166, no. 21 (November 27, 2006).

U.S. Environmental Protection Agency. "Organophosphorus Cumulative Risk Assessment—2006 Update." August 2006. http://www.epa.gov/pesticides/cumulative/2006-op/op_cra_appendices_part1.pdf.

van Birgelen, A., et al. "Synergistic Effect of 2,2',4,4',5,5'-Hexachlorobiphenyl and 2,3,7,8-Tetrachlorodibenzo-p-dioxin on Hepatic Porphyrin Levels in the Rat." *Environmental Health Perspectives* 104, no. 5 (May 1996).

CHAPTER 5

Ahmed, T., et al. "Interleukin-6 Inhibits Growth Hormone–Mediated Gene Expression in Hepatocytes." *American Journal of Physiology: Gastrointestinal and Liver Physiology* 292, no. 6 (June 2007).

Asami, D., et al. "Comparison of the Total Phenolic and Ascorbic Acid Content of Freeze-Dried and Air-Dried Marionberry, Strawberry, and Corn Grown Using Conventional, Organic, and Sustainable Agricultural Practices." *Journal of Agriculture and Food Chemistry* 51, no. 5 (February 26, 2003).

Bauer, S. (ed.) *National Geographic Green Guide.* www.thegreenguide.com.

Benbrook, C. "State of the Science Review: Nutritional Superiority of Plant-Based Organic Foods." The Organic Center. www.organic-center.org (March 2008).

Bermudez, O. "Preliminary Data Suggest that Soda and Sweet Drinks Are the Main Source of Calories in American Diet." ScienceDaily.com ("Consumption of Sweet Drinks among American Adults from the NHANES 1999–2000." Abstract # 839.5, *Experimental Biology* 2005). www.sciencedaily.com/releases/2005/05/050527111920.htm.

Blaylock, R. *Excitotoxins: The Taste That Kills.* Santa Fe, NM: Health Press, 1997.

Burckhardt, I., et al. "Green Tea Catechin Polyphenols Attenuate Behavioral and Oxidative Responses to Intermittent Hypoxia." *American Journal of Respiratory and Critical Care Medicine* 177, no. 10 (May 15, 2008).

Carbonaro, M., et al. "Modulation of Antioxidant Compounds in Organic vs. Conventional Fruit (Peach, *Prunus persica* L., and Pear, *Pyrus communis* L.)." *Journal of Agriculture and Food Chemistry* 50, no. 19 (September 11, 2002).

CBS News. "FDA: Too Much Benzene in Some Drinks." May 19, 2006.

Center for Science in the Public Interest. "Chemical Cuisine: A Guide to Food Additives." *Nutrition Action Health Letter,* May 2008.

Consumer Reports staff. "Benzene in Soft Drinks." *Consumer Reports,* October 2006. www.consumerreports.org/cro/food/food-safety/benzene-in-soft-drinks/benzene-10-06/overview/1006_benzene_ov_1.htm.

Dawson, R., et al. "Attenuation of Leptin-Mediated Effects by Monosodium Glutamate–Induced Arcuate Nucleus Damage" (part 1). *American Journal of Physiology* 273, no. 1 (July 1997).

Dhiman, T. "Role of Diet on Conjugated Linoleic Acid Content of Milk and Meat." Suppl. 1, *Journal of Animal Science* 79 (2001).

Dunn, W., Xu, R., and Schwimmer, J. "Modest Wine Drinking and Decreased Prevalence of Suspected Nonalcoholic Fatty Liver Disease." *Hepatology* 47, no. 6 (June 2008).

Environmental Working Group. "A Survey of Bisphenol A in U.S. Canned Foods." March 5, 2007. www.ewg.org/reports/bisphenola.

Erowid. "Caffeine Content of Beverages, Foods and Medications." www.erowid.org/chemicals/caffeine/caffeine_info1.shtml.

Food and Drug Administration. "Butylated Hydroxyanisole (BHA)." Report on Carcinogens, 11th ed., 2005.

Gorman, R. "Faux Food: Where Have All Our Nutrients Gone?" *EatingWell.* www.eatingwell.com/news_views/special_report/faux_food.html.

Jeong, S., et al. "Effects of Butylated Hydroxyanisole on the Development and Functions of Reproductive System in Rats." *Toxicology* 208, no. 1 (March 1, 2005).

Katcher, H., et al. "The Effects of a Whole Grain–Enriched Hypocaloric Diet on Cardiovascular Disease Risk Factors in Men and Women with Metabolic Syndrome." *American Journal of Clinical Nutrition* 87, no. 1 (January 2008).

Lew, J., et al. "Alcohol Consumption and Risk of Breast Cancer in Postmenopausal Women: The NIH-AARP Diet and Health Study." *Proceedings of the 99th Annual Meeting of the American Association for Cancer Research,* April 12–16, 2008, AACR (2008).

Liu, S., et al. "A Prospective Study of Whole-Grain Intake and Risk of Type 2 Diabetes Mellitus in US Women." *American Journal of Public Health* 90, no. 9 (2000).

Lutsey, P., Steffen, L., and Stevens, J. "Dietary Intake and the Development of the

Metabolic Syndrome: The Atherosclerosis Risk in Communities Study." *Circulation* 117, no. 6 (February 12, 2008).

McCann, D., et al. "Food Additives and Hyperactive Behaviour in 3-Year-Old and 8/9-Year-Old Children in the Community: A Randomised, Double-Blinded, Placebo-Controlled Trial." *The Lancet* 370 (2007).

McLaughlin, K. "A New Taste Sensation." *Wall Street Journal* online. www.wsj.com, December 8, 2007.

Mense, S., et al. "Phytoestrogens and Breast Cancer Prevention: Possible Mechanisms of Action." *Environmental Health Perspectives* 116, no. 4 (April 2008).

Meyer, K., et al. "Carbohydrates, Dietary Fiber, and Incident Type 2 Diabetes in Older Women." *American Journal of Clinical Nutrition* 71, no. 4 (2000).

Moskin, J. "Yes, MSG, the Secret Behind the Savor." *New York Times*, March 5, 2008.

Mozaffarian, D., et al. "Trans Fatty Acids and Cardiovascular Disease." *New England Journal of Medicine* 354, no. 15 (April 13, 2006).

Phytochemicals.info. "Phytochemicals." www.phytochemicals.info/phytochemicals/indole-3-carbinol.php.

Pierce, W., et al. "Overeating by Young Obesity-Prone and Lean Rats Caused by Tastes Associated with Low Energy Foods." *Obesity* 15, no. 8 (August 2007).

Shapiro, A., et al. "Fructose-Induced Leptin Resistance Exacerbates Weight Gain in Response to Subsequent High Fat Feeding." *American Journal of Physiology: Regulatory Integrative and Comparative Physiology* (August 13, 2008).

Swithers, S., and Davidson, T. "A Role for Sweet Taste: Calorie Predictive Relations in Energy Regulation by Rats." *Behavioral Neuroscience* 122, no. 1 (February 2008).

Taubes, G. "What If It's All Been a Big Fat Lie?" *New York Times*, July 7, 2002.

Torii, K., et al. "Hypothalamic Control of Amino Acid Appetite." *Annals of the New York Academy of Sciences* 855 (1998).

UK Food Standards Agency. "Survey of Bisphenols in Canned Foods (Number 13/01)." www.food.gov.uk/science/surveillance/fsis2001/bisphenols (March 19, 2001).

USDA. "USDA—Iowa State University Database on the Isoflavone Content of Foods, Release 1.4." April 2007. http://www.ars.usda.gov/SP2UserFiles/Place/12354500/Data/isoflav/isoflav1-4.pdf.

USDA Economic Research Service. "Dietary Assessment of Major Trends in U.S. Food Consumption, 1970–2005 / EIB-33." www.ers.usda.gov/Publications/EIB33/EIB33.pdf (March 2008).

USDA Economic Research Service. "Food Availability Data Set." March 15, 2008. www.ers.usda.gov/Data/FoodConsumption.

Venables, M., et al. "Green Tea Extract Ingestion, Fat Oxidation, and Glucose Tolerance in Healthy Humans." *American Journal of Clinical Nutrition* 87, no. 3 (March 2008).

Yeager, S. "High-Metabolism Diet: Essential Eating Rules That Stoke Your Fat Burn All Day Long." *Prevention*, March 2008.

Yellayi, S., et al. "The Phytoestrogen Genistein Induces Thymic and Immune Changes: A Human Health Concern?" *Proceedings of the National Academy of Sciences* 99, no. 11 (May 28, 2002).

CHAPTER 6

Alba-Roth, J., et al. "Arginine Stimulates Growth Hormone Secretion by Suppressing Endogenous Somatostatin Secretion." *Journal of Clinical Endocrinology and Metabolism* 67, no. 6 (December 1998).

American Chemical Society. "Sustainable Farm Practices Improve Third World Food Production" (press release), January 23, 2006.

American Heart Association. "Make Healthy Food Choices." April 4, 2008. www.americanheart.org/presenter.jhtml?identifier=537.

American Heart Association. "Triglycerides." www.americanheart.org/presenter.jhtml?identifier=4778.

American Institute for Cancer Research. "Foods That Fight Cancer." 2008. www.aicr.org/site/PageServer?pagename=dc_foods_home.

Anderson, J. "Effects of Psyllium on Glucose and Serum Lipid Responses in Men with Type 2 Diabetes and Hypercholesterolemia." *American Journal of Clinical Nutrition* 70, no. 4 (October 1999).

Armanini, D., et al. "Licorice Reduces Serum Testosterone in Healthy Women." *Steroids* 69, no. 11–12 (October–November 2004).

Badrick, E., et al. "The Relationship between Alcohol Consumption and Cortisol Secretion in an Aging Cohort." *Journal of Clinical Endocrinology and Metabolism* 93, no. 3 (March 2008).

Bagga, D., et al. "Effects of a Very Low Fat, High Fiber Diet on Serum Hormones and Menstrual Function: Implications for Breast Cancer Prevention." *Cancer* 76, no. 12 (December 1995).

Banks, W., et al. "Triglycerides Induce Leptin Resistance at the Blood-Brain Barrier." *Diabetes* 53, no. 5 (May 2004).

Barber, D. "Change We Can Stomach." *New York Times* (op-ed), May 11, 2008.

Bauer, S. (ed.) *National Geographic Green Guide.* www.thegreenguide.com.

Beaven, C. "Dose Effect of Caffeine on Testosterone and Cortisol Responses to Resistance Exercise." *International Journal of Sports Nutrition and Exercise Metabolism* 18, no. 2 (April 2008).

Benbrook, C. "State of the Science Review: Nutritional Superiority of Plant-Based Organic Foods." The Organic Center. www.organic-center.org (March 2008).

"Blueberries and Antioxidant Activity." U.S. Highbush Blueberry Council. http://www.blueberry.org.

Bovee, T., et al. "Screening of Synthetic and Plant-Derived Compounds for (Anti)estrogenic and (Anti)androgenic Activities." *Analytical and Bioanalytical Chemistry* 390, no. 4 (February 2008).

Bowen, J., et al. "Appetite Hormones and Energy Intake in Obese Men after Consumption of Fructose, Glucose and Whey Protein Beverages." *International Journal of Obesity* 31, no. 11 (November 2007).

"Broccoli May Undo Diabetes Damage." BBC News, August 5, 2008. news.bbc.co.uk/2/hi/health/7541639.stm.

Calissendorff, J. "Is Decreased Leptin Secretion after Alcohol Ingestion Catecholamine-Mediated?" *Alcohol and Alcoholism* 39, no. 4 (July and August 2004).

Carper, J. "Eat Smart: Garlic." *USA Weekend,* March 31–April 2, 1995.

"Chromium Picolinate." *The Merck Manual of Medical Information.* www.merck.com/mmhe/sec02/ch019/ch019c.html (February 2003).

Collins, K. "Fight Cancer with Dark Green Vegetables: Average Adult Should Eat Three Cups of Produce a Week." MSNBC.com, April 8, 2005. http://www.msnbc.msn.com/id/7421199/.

Consumer Reports. "When It Pays to Buy Organic." February 2006. www.consumerreports.org.

Cummings, D., et al. "Plasma Ghrelin Levels after Diet-Induced Weight Loss or Gastric Bypass Surgery." *New England Journal of Medicine* 346, no. 21 (May 2002).

Curl, C., Fenske, R., and Elgethun, K. "Organophosphorus Pesticide Exposure of Urban and Suburban Preschool Children with Organic and Conventional Diets." *Environmental Health Perspectives* 111, no. 3 (March 2003).

Dalton, L. "Licorice: Root Is Used Worldwide as a Flavor and a Medicine." *Chemical and Engineering News* 80, no. 32 (August 2002).

"DHEA." Medline Plus, January 01, 2008. www.nlm.nih.gov/medlineplus/druginfo/natural/patient-dhea.html.

Ebisch, I., et al. "The Importance of Folate, Zinc and Antioxidants in the Pathogenesis and Prevention of Subfertility." *Human Reproduction Update* 13, no. 2 (March–April 2007).

"Eicosapentaenoic Acid (EPA)." University of Maryland Medical Center. www.umm.edu/altmed/articles/eicosapentaenoic-acid-000301.htm.

Environmental Working Group. "What's the Difference?" ("The Dirty Dozen") www.foodnews.org/methodology.php.

Erdmann, J., et al., "Postprandial Response of Plasma Ghrelin Levels to Various Test Meals in Relation to Food Intake, Plasma Insulin, and Glucose." *Journal of Clinical Endocrinology and Metabolism* 89, no. 6 (June 2004).

Fenwick, G., Heaney, R., and Mullin, W. "Glucosinolates and Their Breakdown Products in Food and Food Plants." *Critical Reviews in Food and Science Nutrition* 18, no. 2 (1983).

Ferrini, R., and Barrett-Connor, E. "Caffeine Intake and Endogenous Sex Steroid Levels in Postmenopausal Women. The Rancho Bernardo Study." *American Journal of Epidemiology* 144, no. 7 (October 1996).

Field, A., et al. "The Relation of Smoking, Age, Relative Weight, and Dietary Intake to Serum Adrenal Steroids, Sex Hormones, and Sex Hormone–Binding Globulin in Middle-aged Men." *Journal of Clinical Endocrinology and Metabolism* 79, no. 5 (November 1994).

Fischer, L., et al. "Clinical Characteristics and Pharmacokinetics of Purified Soy Isoflavones: Multiple-Dose Administration to Men with Prostate Neoplasia." *Nutrition and Cancer* 48, no. 2 (2004).

Ford, E., and Mokdad, A. "Fruit and Vegetable Consumption and Diabetes Mellitus Incidence among U.S. Adults." *Preventive Medicine* 32, no. 1 (2001).

Foster-Schubert, E. "Acyl and Total Ghrelin Are Suppressed Strongly by Ingested Proteins, Weakly by Lipids, and Biphasically by Carbohydrates." *Journal of Endocrinology and Metabolism* 93, no. 5 (May 2008).

Frecka, J., and Mattes, R. "Possible Entrainment of Ghrelin to Habitual Meal Patterns in Humans." *American Journal of Physiology: Gastrointestinal and Liver Physiology* 294, no. 3 (March 2008).

Fung, T., et al. "Whole-Grain Intake and the Risk of Type 2 Diabetes: A Prospective Study in Men." *American Journal of Clinical Nutrition* 76, no. 3 (2002).

Gianoulakis, C., et al. "Effect of Chronic Alcohol Consumption on the Activity of the Hypothalamic-Pituitary-Adrenal Axis and Pituitary Beta-Endorphin as a Function of Alcohol Intake, Age, and Gender." *Alcoholism: Clinical and Experimental Research* 27, no. 3 (March 2003).

Giltay, E., et al. "Docosahexaenoic Acid Concentrations Are Higher in Women Than in Men Because of Estrogenic Effects." *American Journal of Clinical Nutrition* 80, no. 5 (November 2004).

Giovannucci, E., et al. "Intake of Carotenoids and Retinol in Relation to Risk of Prostate Cancer." *Journal of the National Cancer Institute* 87, no. 23 (1995).

Graham-Row, D. "Organic Tomatoes Have More Antioxidants." July 5, 2007. www.newscientist.com.

"Health Benefits of Thai Soup under Study." CNN.com, January 3, 2001. edition. cnn.com/2001/HEALTH/diet.fitness/01/03/thai.soup.index.html.

Heller, R., et al. "Relationship of High Density Lipoprotein Cholesterol with Total and Free Testosterone and Sex Hormone Binding Globulin." *Acta Endocrinologica* 104, no. 2 (October 1983).

Henig, R. "Fat Factors." *New York Times,* August 13, 2006.

Hershey's. "Licorice and Glycyrrhizic Acid." www.hersheys.com/nutrition/licorice. asp.

Higgins, J. "Resistant Starch: Metabolic Effects and Potential Health Benefits." *Journal of AOAC International* 87, no. 3 (May–June 2004).

Higgins, J., et al. "Resistant Starch Consumption Promotes Lipid Oxidation." *Nutrition and Metabolism* 1, no. 1 (October 6, 2004).

Hu, M., and Hee Poh, N. "Dietary Selenium and Vitamin E Affect Adrenal and Brain Dehydroepiandrosterone Levels in Young Rats." *Journal of Nutritional Biochemistry* 9, no. 6 (June 1998).

International Food Information Council. "Functional Foods Fact Sheet: Plant Stanols and Sterols." July 2007. www.ific.org/publications/factsheets/sterolfs.cfm.

Isaacs, S. *The Leptin Boost Diet.* Berkeley, CA: Ulysses Press, 2007.

Kasim-Karakas, S., et al. "Relation of Nutrients and Hormones in Polycystic Ovary Syndrome." *American Journal of Clinical Nutrition* 85, no. 3 (March 2007).

Katz, D. *The Flavor Point Diet.* Emmaus, PA: Rodale, Inc., 2005.

Kelly, G. "Nutritional and Botanical Interventions to Assist with the Adaptation to Stress." *Alternative Medicine Review* 4, no. 4 (August 1999).

Kerstens, M., et al. "Salt Loading Affects Cortisol Metabolism in Normotensive Subjects: Relationships with Salt Sensitivity." *Journal of Clinical Endocrinology and Metabolism* 88, no. 9 (September 2003).

Kokavec, A., and Crowe, S. "The Effect of a Moderate Level of White Wine Consumption on the Hypothalamic-Pituitary-Adrenal Axis before and after a Meal." *Pharmacology Biochemistry and Behavior* 70, no. 2–3 (October–November 2001).

Kovacs, E., et al. "Effects of Green Tea on Weight Maintenance after Body-Weight Loss." *British Journal of Nutrition* 91, no. 3 (March 2004).

Lee, D. "A Strong Dose-Response Relation between Serum Concentrations of Persistent Organic Pollutants and Diabetes: Results from the National Health and Examination Survey 1999–2002." *Diabetes Care* 29, no. 7 (July 2006).

Lee, J., et al. "Omega-3 Fatty Acids for Cardioprotection." *Mayo Clinic Proceedings* 83, no. 3 (March 2008): 324–32.

Ley, R., et al. "Microbial Ecology: Human Gut Microbes Associated with Obesity." *Nature* 444 (7122), December 21, 2006.

Li, X., Ma, Y., and Liu, X. "Effect of the Lycium Barbarum Polysaccharides on Age-Related Oxidative Stress in Aged Mice." *Journal of Ethnopharmacology* 111, no. 3 (May 22, 2007).

Linus Pauling Institute Micronutrient Information Center, Oregon State University. lpi.oregonstate.edu/infocenter/.

Longcope, C., et al. "Diet and Sex Hormone–Binding Globulin." *Journal of Clinical Endocrinology and Metabolism* 85, no. 1 (January 2000).

Louis Warschaw Prostate Cancer Center. "Fruits and Vegetables: General Information." Cedars-Sinai. www.csmc.edu/3425.html.

Lovallo, W., et al. "Caffeine Stimulation of Cortisol Secretion across the Waking

Hours in Relation to Caffeine Intake Levels." *Psychosomatic Medicine* 67, no. 5 (September–October 2005).

Lovallo, W., et al. "Cortisol Responses to Mental Stress, Exercise, and Meals Following Caffeine Intake in Men and Women." *Pharmacology Biochemistry and Behavior* 83, no. 3 (March 2006).

Low, Y., et al. "Phytoestrogen Exposure Is Associated with Circulating Sex Hormone Levels in Postmenopausal Women and Interact with ESR1 and NR1I2 Gene Variants." *Cancer Epidemiology Biomarkers and Prevention* 16, no. 5 (May 2007).

Lu, L., et al. "Decreased Ovarian Hormones during a Soya Diet: Implications for Breast Cancer Prevention." *Cancer Research* 60, no. 15 (August 2000).

Lutgendorf, S., et al. "Effects of Relaxation and Stress on the Capsaicin-Induced Local Inflammatory Response." *Psychosomatic Medicine* 62, no. 4 (July–August 2000).

Lutsey, P., Steffen, L., and Stevens, J. "Dietary Intake and the Development of the Metabolic Syndrome: The Atherosclerosis Risk in Communities Study." *Circulation* 117, no. 6 (February 12, 2008).

"Magnesium." National Institutes of Health Office of Dietary Supplements. ods.od.nih.gov/factsheets/magnesium.asp.

Mahabir, S., et al. "The Effects of Moderate Alcohol Supplementation on Estrone Sulfate and DHEAS in Postmenopausal Women in a Controlled Feeding Study." *Nutrition Journal* 3, no. 1 (September 2004).

Mantzoros, C., et al. "Zinc May Regulate Serum Leptin Concentrations in Humans." *Journal of American College of Nutrition* 17, no. 3 (June 1998).

Markus, C., et al. "The Bovine Protein Alpha-Lactalbumin Increases the Plasma Ratio of Tryptophan to the Other Large Neutral Amino Acids, and in Vulnerable Subjects Raises Brain Serotonin Activity, Reduces Cortisol Concentration, and Improves Mood under Stress." *American Journal of Clinical Nutrition* 71, no. 6 (June 2000).

Martin, A. "Fighting on a Battlefield the Size of a Milk Label." *New York Times,* March 9, 2008.

Mayo Clinic staff. "High-fructose Corn Syrup: Why Is It So Bad for Me?" MayoClinic. com. www.mayoclinic.com/print/high-fructose-corn-syrup/AN01588/METHOD= print (October 24, 2008).

Mayo Clinic staff. "Niacin to Boost Your HDL 'Good' Cholesterol." MayoClinic.com. www.mayoclinic.com/health/niacin/CL00036 (March 28, 2008).

Mayo Clinic staff. "Sodium: Are You Getting Too Much?" MayoClinic.com. www. mayoclinic.com/health/sodium/NU00284 (May 23, 2008).

McArdle, W. *Exercise Physiology: Energy, Nutrition, and Human Performance.* Philadelphia: Lippincott Williams & Wilkins, April 2006.

McDougall, G., and Stewart, D. "The Inhibitory Effects of Berry Polyphenols on Digestive Enzymes." *Biofactors* 23, no. 4 (2005).

Medline Plus. "Omega-3 Fatty Acids, Fish Oil, Alpha-Linolenic Acid." www.nlm. nih.gov/medlineplus/druginfo/natural/patient-fishoil.html (March 1, 2008).

Medline Plus. "Vitamin C." Medline Plus Medical Encyclopedia. www.nlm.nih.gov/ medlineplus/ency/article/002404.htm (January 1, 2007).

Metzgar, K. "Why the Little Sticky Label on Fruit?" *Rural Connections: The Voice of Hawaii's Organiculture* (newsletter, Hawaii Organic Farmers Association, fall 2004).

Milligan, S., et al. "Identification of a Potent Phytoestrogen in Hops (*Humulus lupulus L.*) and Beer." *Journal of Clinical Endocrinology and Metabolism* 84, no. 6 (June 1999).

Mitchell, A., et al. "Ten-Year Comparison of the Influence of Organic and Conventional Crop Management Practices on the Content of Flavonoids in Tomatoes." *Journal of Agriculture and Food Chemistry* 55, no. 15 (July 25, 2007).

Monroe, K., et al. "Dietary Fiber Intake and Endogenous Serum Hormone Levels in Naturally Postmenopausal Mexican American Women: The Multiethnic Cohort Study." *Nutrition and Cancer* 58, no. 2 (July 2007).

Moore, T., et al. "Reduced Susceptibility to Two-Stage Skin Carcinogenesis in Mice with Low Circulating Insulin-Like Growth Factor I Levels." *Cancer Research* 68, no. 10 (May 15, 2008).

Murtaugh, M., et al. "Epidemiological Support for the Protection of Whole Grains against Diabetes." *Proceedings of the Nutrition Society* 62, no. 1 (February 2003).

Myklebust, M., and Wunder, J. "Legumes" and "Soy." Healing Foods Pyramid, University of Michigan Integrative Medicine. www.med.umich.edu/umim/clinical/pyramid/index.htm (2004).

Nagata, C., et al. "Fat Intake Is Associated with Serum Estrogen and Androgen Concentrations in Postmenopausal Japanese Women." *Journal of Nutrition* 135, no. 12 (December 2005).

Nakanishi, Y., et al. "Increase in Terminal Restriction Fragments of Bacteroidetes-Derived 16S rRNA Genes after Administration of Short-Chain Fructooligosaccharides." *Applied and Environmental Microbiology* 72, no. 9 (September 2006).

Núñez, N., et al. "Alcohol Consumption Promotes Body Weight Loss in Melanoma-Bearing Mice." *Alcoholism: Clinical and Experimental Research* 26, no. 5 (May 2002).

Oi, Y., et al. "Garlic Supplementation Increases Testicular Testosterone and Decreases Plasma Corticosterone in Rats Fed a High Protein Diet." *Journal of Nutrition* 131, no. 8 (August 2001).

Parker-Pope, T. "Finding the Best Way to Cook All Those Vegetables." *New York Times,* May 20, 2008.

Pereira, M., et al. "Effect of Whole Grains on Insulin Sensitivity in Overweight Hyperinsulinemic Adults." *American Journal of Clinical Nutrition* 75, no. 5 (May 2002).

Pérez-Matute, P., et al. "Eicosapentaenoic Fatty Acid Increases Leptin Secretion from Primary Cultured Rat Adipocytes: Role of Glucose Metabolism." *American Journal of Physiology—Regulatory, Integrative, and Comparative Physiology* 288, no. 6 (June 2005).

Peyron-Caso, E., et al. "Dietary (n-3) Polyunsaturated Fatty Acids Up-regulate Plasma Leptin in Insulin-Resistant Rats." *Journal of Nutrition* 132, no. 8 (August 2002).

Physicians Committee for Responsible Medicine. "Using Foods Against Menstrual Pain." www.pcrm.org/health/prevmed/menstrual_pain.html.

Physicians for Social Responsibility. "Environmental Endocrine Disruptors: What Health Care Providers Should Know." www.psr.org/site/DocServer/Environmental_Endocrine_Disruptors.pdf.

Pimentel, D. "Environmental, Energetic, and Economic Comparisons of Organic and Conventional Farming Systems." *BioScience* 55, no. 7 (July 2005).

Prentice, R., et al. "Dietary Fat Reduction and Plasma Estradiol Concentration in Healthy Postmenopausal Women." *Journal of the National Cancer Institute* 82, no. 2 (January 1990).

Promberger, A., et al. "Determination of Estrogenic Activity in Beer by Biological and Chemical Means." *Journal of Agricultural and Food Chemistry* 49, no. 2 (February 2001).

Psychology Today staff. "Vitamin C: Stress Buster." *Psychology Today*, April 25, 2003.

Rahman, R. "Garlic and Aging: New Insights into an Old Remedy. *Ageing Research Reviews* 2, no. 1 (January 2003).

Rao, A. "Lycopene, Tomatoes, and the Prevention of Coronary Heart Disease" (symposia, Society for Experimental Biology and Medicine). *Experimental Biology and Medicine* 227 (2002).

Roediger, W., and Babidge, W. "Human Colonocyte Detoxification." *Gut* 41 (December 1997).

Rosenhagen, M., et al. "Elevated Plasma Ghrelin Levels in Night-Eating Syndrome." *American Journal of Psychiatry* 162, no. 4 (April 2005).

Roy, H., and Lundy, S. "Health Benefits of Cruciferous Vegetables." Pennington Nutrition Series: Healthier Lives through Education in Nutrition and Preventive Medicine, no. 21 (2005). www.pbrc.edu/Division_of_Education/pdf/PNS_Cruciferous_Vegetables.pdf.

Salas-Salvadó, J., et al. "The Effect of Nuts on Inflammation." Suppl. 1, *Asia Pacific Journal of Clinical Nutrition* 17 (2008).

Sampson, L., et al. "Flavonol and Flavone Intakes in US Health Professionals." *Journal of the American Dietetic Association* 102, no. 12 (October 2002).

Seeram, N. "Berry Fruits: Compositional Elements, Biochemical Activities, and the Impact of Their Intake on Human Health, Performance, and Disease." *Journal of Agriculture and Food Chemistry* 56, no. 3 (February 13, 2008).

Sierksma, A., et al. "Effect of Moderate Alcohol Consumption on Plasma Dehydroepiandrosterone Sulfate, Testosterone, and Estradiol Levels in Middle-Aged Men and Postmenopausal Women: A Diet-Controlled Intervention Study." *Alcoholism: Clinical and Experimental Research* 28, no. 5 (May 2004).

Sigurjonsdottir, H., et al. "Liquorice in Moderate Doses Does Not Affect Sex Steroid Hormones of Biological Importance Although the Effect Differs between the Genders." *Hormone Research* 65, no. 2 (2006).

Slavin, J. "Dietary Fiber and Body Weight." *Nutrition* 21, no. 3 (March 2005).

Slavin, J. "Why Whole Grains Are Protective: Biological Mechanisms." *Proceedings of the Nutrition Society* 62, no. 1 (February 2003).

"Smart Balance Omega Plus Light Mayonnaise." www.smartbalance.com/Mayonnaise Family.aspx.

Suzanne Dixon. "Food for Thought: The Facts on Fiber." *Progress Newsletter* (newsletter, University of Michigan Comprehensive Cancer Center, winter 2002). www.cancer.med.umich.edu/news/pro09win02.shtml#four.

Taylor, A., et al. "Impact of Binge Eating on Metabolic and Leptin Dynamics in Normal Young Women." *Journal of Clinical Endocrinology and Metabolism* 84, no. 2 (February 1999).

Teff, K., et al. "Dietary Fructose Reduces Circulating Insulin and Leptin, Attenuates Postprandial Suppression of Ghrelin, and Increases Triglycerides in Women." *Journal of Clinical Endocrinology and Metabolism* 89, no. 6 (June 2004).

The George Mateljan Foundation. The World's Healthiest Foods Web sites, whfoods. org and WorldsHealthiestFoods.com.

Tou, J., et al. "Flaxseed and Its Lignan Precursor, Secoisolariciresinol Diglycoside, Affect Pregnancy Outcome and Reproductive Development in Rats." *Journal of Nutrition* 128, no. 111 (November 1998).

Tsuda, T. "Regulation of Adipocyte Function by Anthocyanins; Possibility of Preventing the Metabolic Syndrome." *Journal of Agriculture and Food Chemistry* 56, no. 3 (February 13, 2008).

Tsuda, T., et al. "Microarray Profiling of Gene Expression in Human Adipocytes in Response to Anthocyanins." *Biochemical Pharmacology* 71, no. 8 (April 14, 2006).

Vartan, S. "Happy Eggs: 'Free Range,' 'Cage Free,' 'Organic'—What's the Story?—Eating Right." *E: The Environmental Magazine,* May–June 2003.

Venables, M., et al. "Green Tea Extract Ingestion, Fat Oxidation, and Glucose Tolerance in Healthy Humans." *American Journal of Clinical Nutrition* 87, no. 3 (March 2008).

"Vitamin E." National Institutes of Health Office of Dietary Supplements. ods.od.nih.gov/factsheets/vitamine.asp.

Walter, M., et al. "Controlled Study on the Combined Effect of Alcohol and Tobacco Smoking on Testosterone in Alcohol-Dependent Men." *Alcohol and Alcoholism* 42, no. 1 (January–February 2007).

Wang, C., et al. "Low-Fat High-Fiber Diet Decreased Serum and Urine Androgens in Men." *Journal of Clinical Endocrinology and Metabolism* 90, no. 6 (June 2005).

Wang, Z., et al. "Effects of Dietary Fibers on Weight Gain, Carbohydrate Metabolism, and Gastric Ghrelin Gene Expression in Mice Fed a High-Fat Diet." *Metabolism* 56, no. 12 (December 2007).

Weigle, D., et al. "A High-Protein Diet Induces Sustained Reductions in Appetite, Ad Libitum Caloric Intake, and Body Weight Despite Compensatory Changes in Diurnal Plasma Leptin and Ghrelin Concentrations." *American Journal of Clinical Nutrition* 82, no. 1 (July 2005).

Winnicki, M., et al. "Fish-Rich Diet, Leptin, and Body Mass." *Circulation* 106, no. 3 (July 2002).

Wolff, R. *Bodybuilding 101.* New York: McGraw-Hill Professional, 2003.

World Cancer Research Fund and the American Institute for Cancer Research. "Second Expert Report: Food, Nutrition, Physical Activity and the Prevention of Cancer: A Global Perspective." 2007. www.dietandcancerreport.org.

Wu, A., et al. "Tea and Circulating Estrogen Levels in Postmenopausal Chinese Women in Singapore." *Carcinogenesis* 25, no. 5 (May 2005).

Wu, W., et al. "Estrogenic Effect of Yam Ingestion in Healthy Postmenopausal Women." *Journal of the American College of Nutrition* 24, no. 4 (August 2005).

Wurst, F., et al. "Gender Differences for Ghrelin Levels in Alcohol-Dependent Patients and Differences between Alcoholics and Healthy Controls." *Alcoholism: Clinical and Experimental Research* 31, no. 12 (December 2007).

Xiong, Y., et al. "Short-Chain Fatty Acids Stimulate Leptin Production in Adipocytes through the G Protein–coupled Receptor GPR41." *Proceedings of the National Academy of Sciences* 101, no. 4 (January 27, 2004).

Xue, M. "Activation of NF-E2-related Factor-2 Reverses Biochemical Dysfunction of Endothelial Cells Induced by Hyperglycemia Linked to Vascular Disease." *Diabetes,* August 2008.

Yeager, S. "High-Metabolism Diet: Essential Eating Rules That Stoke Your Fat Burn All Day Long." *Prevention,* March 2008.

"Zinc." National Institutes of Health Office of Dietary Supplements. ods.od.nih.gov/factsheets/cc/zinc.html#food.

CHAPTER 7

Accurso, A. et al. "Dietary Carbohydrate Restriction in Type 2 Diabetes Mellitus and Metabolic Syndrome: Time for a Critical Appraisal." *Nutrition and Metabolism* 5 (April 8, 2008).

American Diabetes Association. "What You Don't Know Could Hurt You." http:// www.diabetes.org (April 17, 2008).

Bakalar, N. "Skipping Cereal and Eggs, and Packing on Pounds." *New York Times,* March 25, 2008.

Blom, W., et al. "Effect of a High-Protein Breakfast on the Postprandial Ghrelin Response." *American Journal of Clinical Nutrition* 83, no. 2 (February 2006).

Bowen, J., Noakes, M., and Clifton, P. "Appetite Regulatory Hormone Responses to Various Dietary Proteins Differ by Body Mass Index Status Despite Similar Reductions in Ad Libitum Energy Intake." *Journal of Clinical Endocrinology and Metabolism* 91, no. 8 (August 2006).

Carlson, O., et al. "Impact of Reduced Meal Frequency without Caloric Restriction on Glucose Regulation in Healthy, Normal-Weight Middle-Aged Men and Women." *Metabolism* 56, no. 12 (December 2007).

Chapelot, D., et al. "Consequence of Omitting or Adding a Meal in Man on Body Composition, Food Intake, and Metabolism." *Obesity* 14, no. 2 (February 2006).

Gardner, C., et al. "Comparison of the Atkins, Zone, Ornish, and LEARN Diets for Change in Weight and Related Risk Factors among Overweight Premenopausal Women: the A to Z Weight Loss Study: A Randomized Trial." *Journal of the American Medical Association* 297, no. 9 (March 7, 2007).

Hamdy, O. "One Year of Follow-Up after Completion of 12 Weeks of Multidisciplinary Diabetes Weight Management Program Using the Why WAIT Intervention Model in Routine Diabetes Practice" (American Diabetes Association's 68th Annual Scientific Sessions, San Francisco, CA, June 7, 2008).

Holmbäck, U., et al. "Endocrine Responses to Nocturnal Eating—Possible Implications for Night Work." *European Journal of Nutrition* 42, no. 2 (April 2003).

International Food Information Council. "2008 Food & Health Survey: Consumer Attitudes toward Food, Nutrition, and Health." May 14, 2008. Council. http:// www.ific.org.

Jenkins, A., et al. "Carbohydrate Intake and Short-Term Regulation of Leptin in Humans." *Diabetologia* 40, no. 3 (March 1997).

Kuzemchak, S. "Outsmart Your Cravings." *Prevention,* February 2008.

Layman, D., et al. "A Reduced Ratio of Dietary Carbohydrate to Protein Improves Body Composition and Blood Lipid Profiles during Weight Loss in Adult Women." *Journal of Nutrition* 133, no. 2 (February 2003).

Leidy, H., Mattes, R., and Campbell, W. "Effects of Acute and Chronic Protein Intake on Metabolism, Appetite, and Ghrelin during Weight Loss." *Obesity* 15, no. 5 (May 2007).

Major, G., et al. "Clinical Significance of Adaptive Thermogenesis." *International Journal of Obesity* 31, no. 2 (February 2007).

Mars, M., et al. "Fasting Leptin and Appetite Responses Induced by a 4-Day 65%-Energy-Restricted Diet." *International Journal of Obesity* 30, no. 1 (January 2006).

Moore, T., et al. "Reduced Susceptibility to Two-Stage Skin Carcinogenesis in Mice with Low Circulating Insulin-Like Growth Factor I Levels." *Cancer Research* 68, no. 10 (May 15, 2008).

Nakanishi, Y., et al. "Increase in Terminal Restriction Fragments of Bacteroidetes-Derived 16S rRNA Genes after Administration of Short-Chain Fructooligosaccharides." *Applied and Environmental Microbiology* 72, no. 9 (September 2006).

Nielsen, J., and Joensson, E. "Low-Carbohydrate Diet in Type 2 Diabetes: Stable Improvement of Bodyweight and Glycemic Control During 44 Months Follow-Up." *Nutrition and Metabolism* 5, no. 1 (May 22, 2008).

Ruidavets, J., et al. "Eating Frequency and Body Fatness in Middle-Aged Men." *International Journal of Obesity and Related Metabolic Disorders* 26, no. 11 (November 2002).

Simeon Margolis, S. (ed.) "No More Big Macs on New American Plate." www.mercksource.com/pp/us/cns/cns_health_a_to_z.jspzQzpgzEzzSzppdocszSzusz SzcnszSzcontentzSzatozzSzalert10262000zPzhtmlzAztcode=J0724.

The George Mateljan Foundation. The World's Healthiest Foods Web sites, whfoods.org and WorldsHealthiestFoods.com.

Timlin, M., et al. "Breakfast Eating and Weight Change in a 5-Year Prospective Analysis of Adolescents: Project EAT (Eating Among Teens)." *Pediatrics* 121, no. 3 (March 2008).

Wansink, B. *Mindless Eating.* New York: Bantam Dell, 2006.

Westerterp-Plantenga, M., et al. "High Protein Intake Sustains Weight Maintenance after Body Weight Loss in Humans." *International Journal of Obesity and Related Metabolic Disorders* 28, no. 1 (January 2004).

Yeager, S. "High-Metabolism Diet: Essential Eating Rules That Stoke Your Fat Burn All Day Long." *Prevention,* March 2008.

CHAPTER 8

Alonso-Magdalena, P., et al. "The Estrogenic Effect of Bisphenol-A Disrupts the Pancreatic β-Cell Function *In Vivo* and Induces Insulin Resistance." *Environmental Health Perspectives* 114 (2006).

American Chemical Society. "Sustainable Farm Practices Improve Third World Food Production" (press release, January 23, 2006).

American Physiological Society. "Anticipating a Laugh Reduces Our Stress Hormones, Study Shows." *ScienceDaily,* April 10, 2008. www.sciencedaily.com/releases/2008/04/080407114617.htm.

Associated Press. "Irregular Sleep Tied to Obesity, Other Health Problems." *USA Today,* May 7, 2008. www.usatoday.com/news/health/2008-05-07-sleep-obesity_N.htm.

Barber, D. "Change We Can Stomach." *New York Times* (op-ed), May 11, 2008.

Bauer, S. (ed.) *National Geographic Green Guide.* www.thegreenguide.com.

Bergsrud, F., Seelig, B., and Derickson, R. "Treatment Systems for Household Water Supplies: Reverse Osmosis." AE-1047, North Dakota Extension Service, June 1992. www.ag.ndsu.edu/pubs/h2oqual/watsys/ae1047w.htm.

Berk, L., et al. "Modulation of Neuroimmune Parameters during the Eustress of Humor-Associated Mirthful Laughter." *Alternative Therapies in Health and Medicine* 7, no. 2 (March 2001).

Betts, K. "When Chlorine + Antimicrobials = Unintended Consequences." *Environmental Science and Technology,* April 6, 2005.

Bräuner, E., et al. "Indoor Particles Affect Vascular Function in the Aged: An Air Filtration–based Intervention Study." *American Journal of Respiratory and Critical Care Medicine* 177, no. 4 (February 2008).

Brody, J. "You Name It, and Exercise Helps It." *New York Times,* April 29, 2008.

Brunner, E., et al. "Prospective Effect of Job Strain on General and Central Obesity in the Whitehall II Study." *American Journal of Epidemiology* 165, no. 7 (April 1, 2007).

Burdge, G., and Wootton, S. "Conversion of Alpha-Linolenic Acid to Eicosapentaenoic, Docosapentaenoic and Docosahexaenoic Acids in Young Women." *British Journal of Nutrition* 88, no. 4 (October 2002).

Center for Bioenvironmental Research, Tulane and Xavier Universities. "E.hormone: Your Gateway to the Environment and Your Hormones." www.e.hormone.tulane .edu.

Christos, S., et al. "Zinc May Regulate Serum Leptin Concentrations in Humans." *Journal of the American College of Nutrition* 17, no. 3 (June 1998).

Church, T., et al. "Effects of Different Doses of Physical Activity on Cardiorespiratory Fitness among Sedentary, Overweight or Obese Postmenopausal Women with Elevated Blood Pressure: A Randomized Controlled Trial." *Journal of the American Medical Association* 297, no. 19 (May 2007).

Ciloglu, F., et al. "Exercise Intensity and Its Effects on Thyroid Hormones." *Neuroendocrinology Letters* 26, no. 6, (December 2005).

"Clouds in Your Coffee? Try Less Styro, More Foam: Polystyrene Foam Cups & Containers, Styrene Migration, and Your Health." April 08, 2008. www.grinning planet.com/2008/04-08/foam-cups-polystyrene-cups-article.htm.

Cox, L. "Lack of Deep Sleep May Up Diabetes Risk." ABCNews.com, December 31, 2007. www.abcnews.go.com/Health/DiabetesResource/story?id=4069909&page=1.

Dobbs, D. "A Musician Who Performs with a Scalpel." *New York Times,* May 20, 2008.

Elmadfa, I., et al. "The Thiamine Status of Adult Humans Depends on Carbohydrate Intake." *International Journal for Vitamin and Nutrition Research* 71, no. 4 (July 2001).

Environmental Defense Fund. "How Safe Are Fish Oil Supplements?" www.edf. org/page.cfm?tagID=19376.

Environmental Working Group. "A National Assessment of Tap Water Quality." December 20, 2005. www.ewg.org/tapwater/findings.php.

Field, T. "Massage Therapy Effects." *American Psychological Association* 53, no. 12 (1998).

Field, T., et al. "Bulimic Adolescents Benefit from Massage Therapy." *Adolescence* 33, no. 131 (fall 1998).

Flier, J., and Elmquist, J. "A Good Night's Sleep: Future Antidote to the Obesity Epidemic?" *Annals of Internal Medicine* 141, no. 11 (December 7, 2004).

Geddes, L., "Insecticides in Pet Shampoo May Trigger Autism." NewScientist.com, May 15, 2008. www.newscientist.com/channel/health/dn13905-insecticides-in-pet-shampoo-may-trigger-autism.html.

Grewen, K., et al. "Effects of Partner Support on Resting Oxytocin, Cortisol, Norepinephrine, and Blood Pressure before and after Warm Partner Contact." *Psychosomatic Medicine* 67 (2005).

Hamdy, O. "One Year of Follow-Up after Completion of 12 Weeks of Multidisciplinary Diabetes Weight Management Program Using the Why WAIT Intervention Model in Routine Diabetes Practice" (American Diabetes Association's 68th Annual Scientific Sessions, San Francisco, CA, June 7, 2008).

Heilbronn, L., et al. "Effect of 6-Month Calorie Restriction on Biomarkers of Longevity, Metabolic Adaptation, and Oxidative Stress in Overweight Individuals." *Journal of the American Medical Association* 295, no. 13 (April 5, 2006).

Hernandez-Reif, M., et al. "Premenstrual Syndrome Symptoms Are Relieved by Massage Therapy." *Journal of Psychosomatic Obstetrics and Gynecology* 21 (2000).

International Obesity TaskForce. "Endocrine Disruptors in Common Plastics Linked to Obesity Risk." *ScienceDaily,* May 15, 2008, May 22, 2008. www.sciencedaily. com/releases/2008/05/080514091427.htm.

Isaacs, S. *Hormonal Balance.* Boulder, CO: Bull Publishing Company, 2007.

Jaret, P. "A Healthy Mix of Rest and Motion." *New York Times,* May 3, 2007.

Johnston, D., and Master, K. *Green Remodeling*. Gabriola Island, BC, Canada: New Society Publishers, 2004.

Kaiser, J. "Just How Dangerous Is Bisphenol-A?" *ScienceNow Daily News,* April 16, 2008.

Kummer, C. *The Joy of Coffee: The Essential Guide to Buying, Brewing, and Enjoying* (revised and updated). New York: Houghton Mifflin, August 2003.

Light, K. "More Frequent Partner Hugs and Higher Oxytocin Levels Are Linked to Lower Blood Pressure and Heart Rate in Premenopausal Women." *Biological Psychology* 69, no. 1 (2005).

Linus Pauling Institute Micronutrient Information Center, Oregon State University. www.lpi.oregonstate.edu/infocenter/.

Liu, X., et al. "Preliminary Study of the Effects of Tai Chi and Qigong Medical Exercise on Indicators of Metabolic Syndrome and Glycemic Control in Adults with Raised Blood Glucose Levels." *British Journal of Sports Medicine* (April 2, 2008).

Lowry, C. A., et al. "Identification of an Immune-Responsive Mesolimbocortical Serotonergic System: Potential Role in Regulation of Emotional Behavior." *Neuroscience* 146, no. 2 (May 2007).

Lutter, M., et al. "The Orexigenic Hormone Ghrelin Defends against Depressive Symptoms of Chronic Stress." *Nature Neuroscience* 11, no. 7 (July 2008).

Maglione-Garves, C., and Kravitz, L., et al. "Cortisol Connection: Tips on Managing Stress and Weight." www.unm.edu/~lkravitz/Article%20folder/stresscortisol.html.

Major, G., et al. "Clinical Significance of Adaptive Thermogenesis." *International Journal of Obesity* 31, no. 2 (February 2007).

Maleskey, G., and Kittel, M. "Turn On Your Weight Loss Hormones!" *Prevention,* January 2002.

McRandle, P. "Plastic Water Bottles: Green Guide 101." *National Geographic Green Guide,* March/April 2004. www.thegreenguide.com/doc/101/plastic.

McRee, L. "Using Massage and Music Therapy to Improve Postoperative Outcomes." *Association of periOperative Registered Nurses Journal,* September 2003.

Miao, Y., et al. "Folic Acid Prevents and Partially Reverses Glucocorticoid-Induced Hypertension in the Rat." *American Journal of Hypertension* 20, no. 3 (March 2007).

Miyawaki, J., et al. "Perinatal and Postnatal Exposure to Bisphenol A Increases Adipose Tissue Mass and Serum Cholesterol Level in Mice." *Journal of Atherosclerosis and Thrombosis* 14, no. 5 (October 2007).

National Sleep Foundation. "2008 Sleep in America Poll." March 2008. www.sleep foundation.org/site/c.hulXKjM0IxF/b.3933533/.

Pelletier, C., Imbeault, P. and Tremblay, A. "Energy Balance and Pollution by Organochlorines and Polychlorinated Biphenyls." *Obesity Reviews* 4, no. 1 (February 2003).

Physicians for Social Responsibility. "Environmental Endocrine Disruptors: What Health Care Providers Should Know." www.psr.org/site/DocServer/Environmental_Endocrine_Disruptors.pdf.

"Poison Exposures in the United States." National Capital Poison Center. http://www.poison.org/prevent/documents/poison%20stats.pdf.

Prevention staff. "Beauty Sleep: How to Make the Most of Skin's Downtime and Wake Up with a New Glow." www.prevention.com/cda/article/beauty-sleep/3decd08f88803110VgnVCM20000012281eac_/lifelong.beauty/anti.aging.arsenal/skin.care (September 8, 2006).

Rayssiguier, Y., et al. "High Fructose Consumption Combined with Low Dietary Magnesium Intake May Increase the Incidence of the Metabolic Syndrome by Inducing Inflammation." *Magnesium Research* 19, no. 4 (December 2006).

Royte, E. *Bottlemania: How Water Went on Sale and Why We Bought It.* New York: Bloomsbury USA, 2008.

Sadler, J. "Is Bottled Water Any Better Than Tap Water?" Newswise release, April 14, 2008.

Scarth, J., et al. "Modulation of the Growth Hormone-Insulin-Like Growth Factor (GH-IGF) Axis by Pharmaceutical, Nutraceutical and Environmental Xenobiotics: An Emerging Role for Xenobiotic-Metabolizing Enzymes and the Transcription Factors Regulating Their Expression." *Xenobiotica* 36, no. 2–3 (February–March 2006).

Spiegel, K., et al. "Brief Communication: Sleep Curtailment in Healthy Young Men Is Associated with Decreased Leptin Levels, Elevated Ghrelin Levels, and Increased Hunger and Appetite." *Annals of Internal Medicine* 141, no. 11 (December 7, 2004).

Steenhuysen, J. "Formaldehyde Exposure Linked with ALS in U.S. Study." Reuters, April 16, 2008.

Stein, R. "Scientists Finding Out What Losing Sleep Does to a Body." *Washington Post,* October 9, 2005.

"Surprising Advice for Insomniacs: Sleep Less." *Harvard HealthBeat,* May 8, 2008.

Suzawa, M., and Ingraham, H. "The Herbicide Atrazine Activates Endocrine Gene Networks via Non-Steroidal NR5A Nuclear Receptors in Fish and Mammalian Cells." *PLoS ONE* 3, no. 5 (May 2008).

Szabo, L. "Endocrine Disruptor Won't Be on the Label." *USA Today,* October 30, 2007.

Tasali, E., et al. "Slow-Wave Sleep and the Risk of Type 2 Diabetes in Humans." *Proceedings of the National Academy of Sciences* 105, no. 3 (January 2008).

The George Mateljan Foundation. The World's Healthiest Foods Web sites, whfoods.org and WorldsHealthiestFoods.com.

Tremblay, A., et al. "Thermogenesis and Weight Loss in Obese Individuals: A Primary Association with Organochlorine Pollution." *International Journal of Obesity and Related Metabolic Disorders* 28, no. 7 (July 2004).

Tugend, A. "Shortcuts: Vacations Are Good for You, Medically Speaking." *New York Times,* June 7, 2008.

University of Maryland Medical Center Complementary and Alternative Medicine Index (CAM). http://www.umm.edu/altmed/.

Volek, J., et al. "Testosterone and Cortisol in Relationship to Dietary Nutrients and Resistance Exercise." *Journal of Applied Physiology* 82, no. 1 (January 1997).

Weinhold, B. "Pollutants May Put On the Pounds." *Environmental Health Perspectives* 114, no. 12 (December 2006).

Whittelsey, F. "Hazards of Hydration." *Sierra,* November–December 2003.

World Cancer Research Fund and the American Institute for Cancer Research. "Second Expert Report: Food, Nutrition, Physical Activity and the Prevention of Cancer: A Global Perspective." 2007. www.dietandcancerreport.org.

Xue, M. "Activation of NF-E2-related Factor-2 Reverses Biochemical Dysfunction of Endothelial Cells Induced by Hyperglycemia Linked to Vascular Disease." *Diabetes,* August 2008.

Yeager, S. "High-Metabolism Diet: Essential Eating Rules That Stoke Your Fat Burn All Day Long." *Prevention,* March 2008.

Zandonella, C. "The Bisphenol-A Debate: A Suspect Chemical in Plastic Bottles and Cans." *National Geographic Green Guide,* May–June 2006. www.thegreenguide. com/doc/114/bpa.

CHAPTER 10

Bell, G., et al. "End-Organ Responses to Thyroxine Therapy in Subclinical Hypothyroidism." *Clinical Endocrinology* 22, no. 1 (January 1985).

Feldman, H. "Age Trends in the Level of Serum Testosterone and Other Hormones in Middle-Aged Men: Longitudinal Results from the Massachusetts Male Aging Study." *Journal of Clinical Endocrinology and Metabolism* 87 (2) (February 2002).

Hernandez-Reif, M., et al. "Premenstrual Syndrome Symptoms Are Relieved by Massage Therapy." *Journal of Psychosomatic Obstetrics and Gynecology* 21 (britannica .com 2000).

Houston, D., et al. "Dietary Protein Intake Is Associated with Lean Mass Change in Older, Community-Dwelling Adults: The Health, Aging, and Body Composition (Health ABC) Study," *American Journal of Clinical Nutrition* 87, no. 1 (January 2008): 150–55.

Mayo Clinic staff. "Lose a Little; Helps a Lot." *Mayo Clinic Health Letter,* January 2008.

Shores, M. "Low Serum Testosterone and Mortality in Male Veterans." *Archives of Internal Medicine* 166, no. 15 (August 14–28, 2006).

"Studies Support Testosterone Supplements for Older Men: Low Levels of the Hormone Could Boost Death Risk, Researchers Say." *U.S. News & World Report,* June 17, 2008. health.usnews.com/articles/health/healthday/2008/06/17/studies-support-testosterone-supplements-for.html.

The Merck Manual of Medical Information. www.merck.com/mmhe/index.html.

U.S. Environmental Protection Agency. "Lindane Voluntary Cancellation and RED Addendum Fact Sheet." July 2006. www.epa.gov/oppsrrd1/REDs/factsheets/lindane_fs_addendum.htm.

Vigorito, C., et al. "Beneficial Effects of a Three-Month Structured Exercise Training Program on Cardiopulmonary Functional Capacity in Young Women with Polycystic Ovary Syndrome." *Journal of Clinical Endocrinology and Metabolism* 92, no. 4 (April 2007).

INDEX

JILLIAN MICHAELS AND BODYMEDIA FIT
ARE THE PERFECT COMBINATION

The Jillian Michaels 360° Weight Loss Navigator™ combines BodyMedia®'s sophisticated data capturing technology with the benefits of a JillianMichaels.com subscription to give you all of the tools you need for a healthier life. Wear your Armband to track your calorie burn, steps taken, and sleep quality. Then, simply log onto JillianMichaels.com to sync your data and access all of the support, recipes, exercises and advice from ME! Best of all, get daily nutritional & fitness feedback based on your goals, progress, and body metrics.

"My 360° WLN program is the ULTIMATE weight-loss system. The program is a total wellness solution designed to get you in the best shape of your life!"

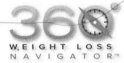

Program comes with:

- BodyMedia FIT Armband and Activity Manager*
- Daily Feedback from ME
- Customized cardio and fitness planner
- 1,000+ recipes
- Community Message Boards

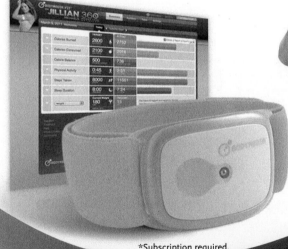

*Subscription required.

BODYMEDIA | FIT™

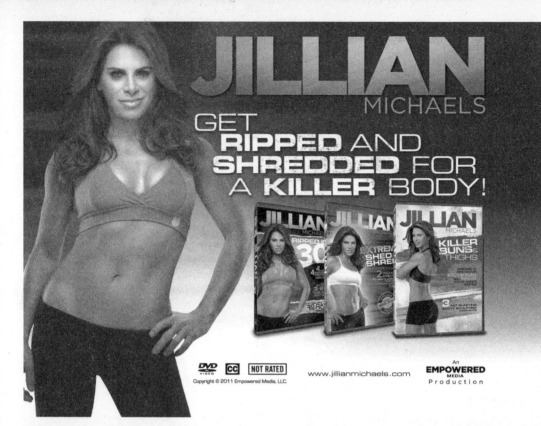
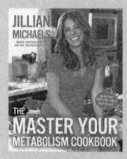
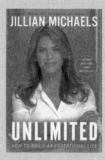
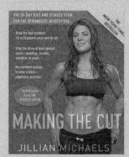